KU-378-217

What To Eat
When You're
Pregnant

Including *the* A–Z of what's safe and what's not

Dr Rana Conway

PEARSON
Prentice Hall
LIFE

Harlow, England • London • New York • Boston • San Francisco • Toronto • Sydney • Singapore • Hong Kong
Tokyo • Seoul • Taipei • New Delhi • Cape Town • Madrid • Mexico City • Amsterdam • Munich • Paris • Milan

Pearson Education Limited

Edinburgh Gate
Harlow CM20 2JE
Tel: +44 (0)1279 623623
Fax: +44 (0)1279 431059
Website: www.pearsoned.co.uk

First published in Great Britain in 2008

ISBN: 978-0-273-71699-0

British Library Cataloguing-in-Publication Data
A catalogue record for this book is available from the British Library

Library of Congress Cataloging-in-Publication Data
Conway, Rana
 What to eat when you're pregnant : including the A-Z of what's safe and what's not / Rana Conway.
    p. cm.
 Includes bibliographical references and index.
 ISBN 978-0-273-71699-0 (alk. paper)
 1. Pregnancy --Nutritional aspects. I. Title.
 RG559.C665 2008
 618.2'42--dc22
                          2008024949

We are grateful to the following for permission to reproduce copyright material: Table 1.1 from *Nutrition During Pregnancy*, Washington, DC, National Academies Press (Institute of Medicine 1990). Reprinted with permission from the National Academies Press, Copyright 1990, National Academy of Sciences; Crown Copyright material is reproduced with the permission of the Controller of HMSO and the Queen's Printer for Scotland.

10 9 8 7 6 5 4 3 2 1
12 11 10 09 08

Typeset in 9.5/13pt Apex by 30
Printed in Great Britain by Henry Ling Ltd., at the Dorset Press, Dorchester, Dorset

The publisher's policy is to use paper manufactured from sustainable forests.

To my three beautiful babies –
Joseph, Daniel and Madeleine

Contents

About the author

Rana Conway (BSc, PhD, RPHNutr) has been a nutritionist for more than 15 years. She has carried out research at leading universities and established herself as an expert in nutrition for pregnancy and childhood. She is *Practical Parenting* magazine's Food Doctor and also writes for the NCT. Her first book *Meals Without Tears: How to Get Your Child to Eat Healthily and Happily* was published in 2007. She has three young children.

Acknowledgements

A big thank you to Rachael Stock, Emma Shackleton and Emma Easy who expertly got this book into shape, and to Jane Graham Maw and Jennifer Christie for all their help.

Also, thank you to everyone else who provided me with help and advice: Dr Adrienne Cullum (NICE), Adam Hardgrave and Olu Adetokunbo (Food Standards Agency), Iain Gillespie (Health Protection Agency), Deb Futers (Professional Lead: Health Visiting, South Staffordshire PCT), Fiona Ford (Centre for Pregnancy Nutrition, University of Sheffield), Carol Key (Customer Services, Sainsbury's), Abigail Enaburekhan (Customer Services, Tesco) and Olly Conway (editorial, computer and emotional support and husband).

Introduction

The food and drink you consume during pregnancy can have an enormous impact on the health and development of your baby. It also plays a crucial role in keeping you fit and well, at a time when your body is working especially hard. Eating regularly and having a well-balanced and varied diet is more important now than ever. But don't worry: this doesn't mean you have to follow a special strict diet or eat specific foods that you generally avoid. You just have to think about your diet a bit more. Start by working out which healthier foods you actually enjoy and would eat regularly – it's important to be realistic when planning any changes to your diet, otherwise you will find it hard to stick to them. This book will show you how you can eat well without too much fuss. If the merest whiff of fish turns your stomach, or the thought of milk makes you grimace, it will point you towards alternative sources of omega 3s or calcium. Eating well should be enjoyable, not an ordeal.

As you read the chapters on healthy eating and essential nutrients, you will see that the best diet for pregnancy is not as complicated as you might think. This book identifies which foods are great for your growing baby and which ones you should try to avoid. It also explains how diet can be used to tackle common problems such as morning sickness, how to achieve a healthy weight gain and what to look out for if you are vegetarian. It should allay any fears you have and leave you feeling confident that you are doing the best for your baby. It also covers what to eat while breastfeeding, and the ideal diet to follow when you start thinking about your next baby. (If you are reading this book in anticipation of getting pregnant, then this final chapter is the best place to begin.) Whatever your stage of pregnancy, once you know you are doing the very best for your baby and avoiding any problem foods, it will help you to enjoy your pregnancy to the full.

Most women get plenty of general advice about healthy eating for pregnancy, but they do not all get enough answers to specific questions. If you are worrying about exactly which cheeses should be avoided or whether peanuts are OK, you'll find the answers here. The A–Z of foods means you can look up anything you're not sure about to discover whether it's safe to eat.

On the other hand, some women find they get too much conflicting advice, which can be overwhelming. To help anybody who is unsure about what to take seriously and what to ignore, we begin by looking at the most common questions and myths.

Common questions

Everyone disagrees about what you can eat. Who can I trust?

Most people agree on what makes up a healthy diet during pregnancy (fruit and vegetables, iron-rich foods, etc.). But when it comes to what to avoid, confusion reigns. Women are bombarded with advice from doctors and midwives, friends and family, magazines, books, supermarkets and websites. And what you are told may be 30 years out of date, or relate to other countries where the food poisoning risks are different.

The Food Standards Agency (FSA) is an independent government department responsible for providing information and advice about healthy eating in the UK. Its guidelines are updated regularly and based on sound evidence. They are often referred to by other organisations such as the Royal College of Midwives, the British Nutrition Foundation and NCT (formerly the National Childbirth Trust). The National Institute for Health and Clinical Excellence (NICE) has also published guidance on maternal and child nutrition.

Sometimes women are given advice by their doctor or midwife that goes against the latest guidelines from the FSA or NICE. This is more likely to be because the doctor or midwife hasn't had enough time to investigate the latest recommendations, rather than a genuine difference of opinion. Internet chat rooms can be another source of conflicting advice: they may provide valuable support and a sense of camaraderie, but you should be careful about following suggestions that are not backed by experts. Frequently, women post messages such as 'I craved ripe Brie and ate it all the time I was expecting my son. He was a healthy 9lb baby, so soft cheese can't really be that bad!' or 'My homeopath told me to stop having dairy foods while I was breastfeeding and it cured my son's colic completely.' Such messages are, no doubt, well meant, but they don't prove anything. Most of us have heard about people who smoked 40 cigarettes a day and lived to 90, but we don't do it ourselves. Reports from individuals can be very compelling, but it is more sensible to follow advice based on the experiences of large numbers of women. The FSA and NICE offer such advice.

Sometimes there are genuine differences of opinion, because clear evidence regarding the safety or health benefits of a particular food or diet is not available. The most controversial areas at the moment are alcohol and caffeine. There is also some debate about how much oily fish should be eaten, and whether or not women should avoid eating peanuts while pregnant or breastfeeding. When the findings of a new study are reported, it is crucial to consider them in the context of all the other available evidence and not to go on the media's interpretation.

How does the government decide what is safe?

When advising pregnant women about which foods are safe and healthy, expert groups such as the FSA and NICE take into account the best evidence available around the world. For example, when assessing how much oily fish you can eat, they will look at investigations into the relationship between fish consumption and birth weight. They will also use their experience of how the UK food industry works and look at data on food safety issues, such as surveys monitoring salmonella contamination in eggs.

Eating food, like crossing the road, or just about any other activity, carries some risk. Any food could be potentially dangerous. In recent years, there have been cases of listeria and salmonella contamination in products as diverse as sandwiches and chocolate. Pregnant women are advised to avoid a particular food only if it has consistently been found to pose a risk to health and the consequences of eating it are thought to be significant. By taking into account all the evidence, it is possible to balance information about health benefits against potential risks for foods such as oily fish, blue cheese or pâté.

I feel so sick I can't even look at fruit or vegetables. How will it affect my baby?

It doesn't seem fair does it? Just when you've resolved to eat a model diet for two, morning sickness (or morning, noon and night sickness) strikes and you have to re-think. This is quite normal. Feelings of nausea or sickness affect about three-quarters of women in early pregnancy.

The good news is that, although you are feeling awful, your baby is very unlikely to be affected. Research shows that mothers who suffer from pregnancy sickness are just as likely to have healthy babies as those who don't. If you are not eating very much or not keeping very much down, your baby will simply draw on your store of nutrients. If you can't face proper meals, then eating small snacks throughout the day will help to keep up your strength. Ideally you should make snacks as healthy as possible (see pages 8–9), but if you can't face anything other than salty crisps or fruit pastilles, then don't worry. Just try to eat more healthily as soon as you start feeling a bit better. There are lots of things you can do to help relieve your symptoms, and make yourself feel more normal, so why not give some of them a try (see page 59)?

I got really drunk before I knew I was pregnant. Will my baby be damaged?

If you drank a lot of alcohol before finding out you were pregnant, try to relax. You are certainly not the first woman to do this, and you won't be the last. There is very little chance that one or two nights of heavy drinking early on in pregnancy will cause any harm. Although drinking alcohol in pregnancy does increase the chances of problems, it in no way makes them a certainty. Worrying or feeling guilty about what has happened won't help. However, once you suspect you are pregnant, it is best to stick to the advice for drinking alcohol in pregnancy (see page 26).

What should I do if I eat something I shouldn't have?

If you eat something and later find out it is on the 'avoid list', try to keep things in perspective. If you feel OK, then try not to worry. The chances of getting food poisoning on any single occasion are extremely small. Instead, remember that stress can have adverse affects on a developing baby, so try to relax and be glad you are not feeling sick.

If you do feel unwell, then it may be a coincidence or a result of something else, such as morning sickness, but go to your doctor as soon as possible. He or she will be able to assess whether you might have listeria, salmonella or any other form of food poisoning. If necessary, your doctor can arrange for you to be tested and, if the tests prove positive, for you to receive treatment to avoid the infection passing to your baby.

I've never heard of anyone getting listeria or toxoplasmosis. Isn't the advice overcautious?

The chances of you getting any form of food poisoning are very small. However, you are more likely to get sick from something you eat when you are pregnant than when you are not pregnant. This is because your immune system undergoes several changes so your body doesn't reject your growing baby. It is estimated that during pregnancy, you are about 20 times more likely than usual to get listeriosis.

Although you may not personally know anyone who has been affected by anything she has eaten during pregnancy, there are cases every year in the UK. According to the baby charity Tommy's, 65 babies are affected by toxoplasmosis each year in the UK. The most common cause of infection is eating cured or undercooked meat. There are also some 20 to 25 cases of listeriosis in pregnant women each year, according to the Health Protection Agency (HPA). The numbers are small, but when you consider that infection could result in miscarriage or stillbirth, you can understand why women are advised to avoid particular foods during pregnancy. Ultimately it is up to the individual to assess whether any risk is worth taking.

Common myths about eating and drinking in pregnancy

Myths and old wives' tales about pregnancy abound. Some are repeated so often in the media, even now, that it's hard to know what to believe and what really is just a myth.

Pregnant women should eat for two

There is some truth in this one. What you eat and drink now will affect both you and your baby. However, if you take it to mean that you need to eat twice as much as usual, then this certainly isn't the case. Sorry to spoil any dreams you have of lying around eating chocolates. Current recommendations suggest that women don't need to eat any more than usual during the first six months of pregnancy; after that, they need only 200 kcal (0.8 MJ) extra a day. That is equivalent to an extra bowl of cereal, or a pot of yogurt and an apple, or a banana and a digestive biscuit, or one scoop of premium ice cream. It's best to follow your appetite, but also to stick to a healthy diet, and not to use pregnancy as an excuse for getting fat. If you do, you'll have the extra challenge of losing weight on top of looking after a baby.

Women in France are allowed to drink loads of wine when they're pregnant and their babies are fine

In France, as in the USA, Canada, Australia and New Zealand, pregnant women are advised not to drink any alcohol in pregnancy. The French, as a nation of wine drinkers, have traditionally been more relaxed about mums-to-be having the odd tipple, and we still have an image of sophisticated French women with a glass of red. However, in 2006 the French authorities brought in new guidelines recommending total abstinence, based on evidence that moderate levels of drinking were linked with permanent brain damage for the baby.

Some pregnant women in France still drink in moderation during pregnancy, but 'moderation' in France probably means less than here in the UK. A pregnant French woman would be very unlikely to drink spirits, and she would have only one small glass of wine with a meal – and then only occasionally. A British woman who drinks 'in moderation' is likely to have much more than this. When the Department of Health advised women to drink only 1 to 2 units once or twice a week, nearly 1 in 10 pregnant women was found to be drinking more. Part of the problem is the British drinking culture. Also, many of us underestimate the number of units of alcohol in our favourite drink (see page 27).

If you eat peanuts, your baby will be allergic to them

The majority of women can enjoy peanuts while they are pregnant or breastfeeding without any worries. Only women with a family history of allergies are currently advised to avoid them. This is the case if you, your baby's father, or any of your other children has food allergies, asthma, eczema or hay fever.

The current government advice dates from 1998 when the Committee on Toxicology (COT) last reviewed the subject. However, the evidence that avoiding peanuts will reduce the risk of your baby developing an allergy now seems, at best, weak. Some believe that early exposure to peanuts isn't the reason why allergies are becoming more common – an alternative theory is that the rise in overclean environments is responsible. Research is now being carried out to see whether normal exposure is in fact better than complete avoidance.

The FSA is currently reviewing the evidence published since 1998, and in 2009 the government may bring out new guidelines. However, as the jury is still out, and with 1 in 70 children now affected by a peanut allergy, which in severe cases can result in anaphylactic shock that can be life-threatening, avoidance is still recommended.

If you followed all the advice, you'd end up eating nothing

We love to blame the 'Food Police' for spoiling our fun and making us eat nothing but alfalfa sprouts. However, it is important to keep things in perspective. There is actually very little that is completely off limits when you are pregnant. The foods that make up the bulk of our everyday diets, such as bread, cereals and milk, can still be enjoyed guilt-free, as can occasional treats such as chocolate and chips. Most women find that only some of the advice about what to avoid is relevant to them. You might find, for example, that the advice about pâté and oysters isn't relevant to you because you never eat these anyway, but if your favourite cheese is Stilton you need to find something else, such as a mature Cheddar, to replace it. Or if you are craving Stilton, have it hot.

In most cases, it is fairly easy to find an alternative for the foods, and even the drinks, that you enjoy. A decaf cappuccino can be a fairly good substitute for the real thing. Once you understand more about why pregnant women are advised to avoid certain foods, you will see that there are plenty of tasty foods you can eat, or precautions you can take to make the foods you usually eat safer. For example, eggs are OK, as long as they are cooked properly. And you can use mayonnaise from a jar instead of homemade. If you are still feeling hard done by, remember that it's for a good cause, and it's not forever.

Drinking beer is good for breastfeeding

For centuries, it has been thought that drinking alcohol, particularly beer, can improve the amount and quality of a mother's breast milk. Some claim a scientific basis for this. In the 1980s, research showed that beer increased levels of prolactin (a hormone essential for breastfeeding). However, this effect was found only in men and non-breastfeeding women. More recent research, looking at the levels of prolactin and other important hormones in breastfeeding mothers, found that alcohol negatively affected the overall hormonal balance.

Several studies have now confirmed the finding that beer, and other alcohol, actually reduces milk production. In a study in Pennsylvania, USA, women were given either normal beer or non-alcoholic beer to see how feeding was affected. Over a four-hour period, the babies in both groups spent about the same amount of time breastfeeding, while the mothers said they had experienced a normal letdown of milk and their babies had fed enough. However, weighing the babies after feeding revealed that they consumed significantly less milk when their mothers drank alcoholic beer.

So, it seems that drinking beer, like any other alcoholic drink, while breastfeeding is actually counterproductive for the baby.

1 Healthy eating for two

Healthy eating is never more important than when you are pregnant. Your diet will affect your baby and yourself both now and for years to come. It may even influence your grandchildren's health. In the immediate term, a healthy diet can help prevent constipation and other common pregnancy problems. It will also provide the energy and nutrients your baby needs to grow and develop in the coming months, so he or she has the best start in life. What you eat in pregnancy is also important for your child's long-term health. There is increasing evidence that a mother's diet during pregnancy affects whether her baby has allergies in childhood or develops heart disease in later life.

During pregnancy, your diet needs to supply all your normal energy and nutrient requirements, but it also has to:

- provide all the needs of your growing baby;
- fuel the growth of new tissue, including the breasts, uterus and placenta;
- lay down a store for the final weeks of pregnancy when your baby is growing rapidly and for breastfeeding.

Enough calories for two

The total energy cost of pregnancy is estimated to be around 76000kcal (calories). This is for a healthy woman gaining an average amount of weight. It sounds like a lot, but don't reach for the chocolate biscuits just yet. Changes to your metabolism, and a reduction in exercise and general activity, mean you don't actually need to consume many more calories during pregnancy than you usually do. In fact, for the first six months, women of a healthy pre-pregnancy weight don't need any extra calories at all. Then, during the final three months, they need only an extra 200 calories (0.8MJ) a day. This is the time when the baby is growing rapidly and laying down fat in preparation for birth.

Appetites vary greatly and some women find that they are incredibly hungry at the beginning of pregnancy, even though their baby is no bigger than a raisin. This is due to hormonal changes and the adaptations that the body is already making. Usually this settles down as pregnancy progresses. Energy requirements also vary from person to person according to a variety of factors, including weight and level of physical activity. If you are underweight you may need extra calories from the beginning. It is important to listen to your body but not to use pregnancy as an excuse for overeating.

Early learning

What you eat now can affect your baby for life. In the late 1980s, David Barker and colleagues explored the idea that the risk of developing certain adult diseases, including stroke and type 2 diabetes, was associated with development in the womb. This is sometimes referred to as the 'Barker hypothesis', but many researchers around the world have carried out similar investigations. There is now a considerable amount of evidence showing that babies with lower birth weight are at greater risk of developing coronary heart disease in later life.

The exact reason for this is not known, but it is believed that babies are somehow 'programmed' in the womb. If they are undernourished before birth, then their body adapts, ready for a life of food deprivation. When they are born into an environment where food is actually abundant, their body can't cope. The real problem is the mismatch between the food supply in the womb and their diet outside. The metabolism of these small babies has been set to store fat, particularly around the waist, which increases the risk of heart disease and other conditions.

Allergy-proofing your baby

If you, your baby's father, or any of your other children has allergies, including eczema, asthma or hay fever, you should avoid eating peanuts during pregnancy and while breastfeeding. Otherwise don't worry. In fact, by eating peanuts and exposing your baby to a small amount of peanut proteins, you may even help him or her to become more tolerant and less likely to develop an allergy.

Even if you have a family history of allergies, there is no need to avoid other foods, such as dairy, wheat and eggs. Research suggests that this will not protect your baby from allergies and may mean you both miss out on essential nutrients. However, there is some evidence that you may be able to reduce your baby's risk of developing allergies by adjusting your diet in other ways during pregnancy. A study of more than 2000 pre-school children in the Bristol area looked at the incidence of wheezing and eczema in relation to mineral levels at birth. It was found that these problems were less common among children who had been born with higher levels of **iron** and **selenium**. This was found by analysing blood samples from the umbilical cords, which primarily reflects the mothers' dietary intake. So, ensuring a good intake of iron and selenium could be valuable tools for allergy protection (see pages 45 and 47 to find out where they are found).

Fish oils have also been shown to help in preventing allergic conditions. Australian researchers found that when pregnant women took fish oil supplements, their babies were three times less likely to show signs of egg allergy at one year of age. The researchers had hoped that the supplements might also reduce the incidence of eczema, but this wasn't the case. However, although there were similar numbers of babies with eczema in the fish oil group as in the placebo group, those with mothers who had taken fish oil had significantly milder symptoms.

As well as getting plenty of iron, selenium and fish oils, some **probiotics** and **prebiotics** (see page 103) may also help when it comes to allergy-proofing. In one study, exposure to probiotics before and after birth was found to be protective against eczema. The trial involved Lactobacillus GG, which was given to women with a family history of atopy (allergic conditions) from 36 weeks of pregnancy until delivery. The women's babies then received the probiotic for six months either directly in formula, or via breast milk when the mothers had it. At the ages of 2 and 4 years, children exposed to the probiotic were much less likely to have eczema than those receiving a placebo in the trial. Other studies have found that a combination of several probiotics along with a prebiotic offers similar protection. Some studies have not found a positive effect on immunity from probiotics, and it may be that different strains have different effects, and that dose and timing of exposure are important. Although the interest in probiotics is still relatively new, overall they appear to have positive effects for people with allergies in the family.

Don't let allergy warnings alarm you
There is no need to avoid foods just because they are labelled with 'Allergy information' or 'Allergy advice'. This simply highlights ingredients, such as milk and peanuts, that most commonly cause allergic reactions. This is so that people with allergies to these specific foods don't miss them in a long list of other ingredients.

How to grow a baby

From conception to birth, a baby needs enormous quantities of nutrients to grow. The requirements include about 925g of protein and 20–30g of calcium, as well as a massive 680mg of iron, equivalent to the amount found in about 34kg of beef or 113 cans of baked beans. Fortunately, you don't actually need to consume all these extra nutrients. Just as your body becomes more efficient at using energy, so it gets better at extracting certain nutrients from the food you eat. As pregnancy progresses and you require more iron, so your body absorbs more. In the first three months of pregnancy, women have been found to absorb only 7% of dietary iron, but this increases to 36% around the middle of pregnancy and to 66% by the end. Because of these metabolic changes, your requirements for certain nutrients, including calcium, iron and vitamin B_{12}, are no greater than normal. However, many young women in the UK consume too little of these nutrients anyway, so it is important to ensure you have a good intake now. The requirements for other nutrients, including zinc, thiamine, riboflavin, folate and vitamins A, C and D, are higher during pregnancy.

Although it is essential that you get all these nutrients, you don't need to worry about monitoring your intake of each vitamin and mineral every day. If you eat a healthy and varied diet, full of wholesome unprocessed foods, you should be getting all the nutrients you need. The healthy diet checklist on page 7 shows the different types of food you should be eating and the main nutrients they supply. You can see how a diet including all of these food groups contains all the essential nutrients. If you want to find out more about any particular nutrient, you can look it up in Chapter 3. To get a better idea of how much of your diet should be taken up by different foods, look at the 'eatwell plate' overleaf. Some people are surprised at just how much carbohydrate-rich foods, fruit and vegetables we should be eating.

FOOD STANDARDS AGENCY
food.gov.uk

The eatwell plate

Use the eatwell plate to help you get the balance right. It shows how much of what you eat should come from each food group.

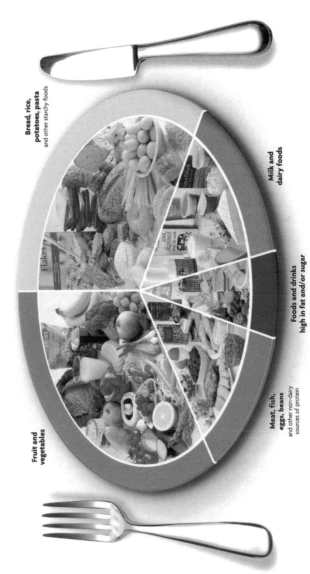

Bread, rice, potatoes, pasta and other starchy foods

Milk and dairy foods

Fruit and vegetables

Meat, fish, eggs, beans and other non-dairy sources of protein

Foods and drinks high in fat and/or sugar

The eatwell plate

Source: Food Standards Agency, http://www.eatwell.gov.uk/healthydiet/eatwellplate/ (last accessed 1 May 2008). © Crown copyright 2007.

The healthy diet checklist

A healthy diet for two should include the following:

- A variety of **fruit and vegetables** (fresh, frozen, tinned or dried). Aim for at least five portions a day for a good supply of vitamins A, C and E, folic acid and iron.

- Plenty of **starchy foods** such as breakfast cereals, bread, rice, pasta and potatoes for carbohydrates, B vitamins and zinc. If you have wholegrain varieties, such as brown rice, you'll also get plenty of fibre to help prevent constipation.

- **Protein foods** such as lean meat, chicken, fish, eggs, beans and lentils. These also supply iron and zinc.

- **Dairy foods** such as milk, cheese and yogurt to provide calcium, vitamin B_{12} and extra protein.

- **Iron-rich foods**, such as meat and fish, green vegetables and fortified breakfast cereals, to prevent anaemia.

- Good sources of **folic acid**, such as oranges, broccoli and fortified breakfast cereals.

- **Oily fish** (once or twice a week) to supply omega 3s for brain and eye development, plus protein, iron and vitamins B_6, B_{12} and D.

Ten ways to boost your fruit and vegetable intake

1 Mix some chopped fruit, such as banana or strawberries, with your breakfast cereal.
2 Have a piece of fruit ready for a mid-morning snack.
3 Keep some raisins, dried apricots, figs or prunes in your desk drawer or handbag ready for when hunger strikes.
4 Add plenty of salad (washed well) to sandwiches.
5 Buy some frozen vegetables. Then, even if you're too tired for peeling and chopping, you can microwave them to go with your evening meal.

6 Make a fruit pudding such as fruit salad, apple crumble or raspberry fool.

7 Mix up a fruit smoothie with bananas, strawberries, blueberries or mangoes.

8 Have some vegetable soup for lunch or make a really chunky soup for supper.

9 Have a glass of pure fruit juice with your evening meal (if you choose a high vitamin-C juice, it'll help iron absorption too).

10 Add extra vegetables when cooking dishes such as shepherd's pie, pasta, fish pie and pizza.

Time for a little something

During pregnancy you are more likely than usual to be rubbing your tummy and looking for a little snack. It may be that you are suffering from morning sickness and can't face proper meals, and so you are trying to eat small amounts rather than nothing. Or perhaps snacking seems the only way to keep nausea at bay. Eating little and often can also be helpful towards the end of pregnancy if you are suffering from heartburn or if large meals just leave you feeling uncomfortable.

When you eat snacks, try to make them as healthy as possible. Avoid always choosing chocolate, biscuits and crisps, as these contain 'empty calories'. This means that they provide energy (calories) but not the essential nutrients, particularly the vitamins and minerals, that you need. Also, research suggests that if you eat a lot of junk food during pregnancy, your baby is likely to turn into a lover of unhealthy food too. So, instead of picking up a fatty or sugary snack, go for something that will provide you with a slower release of energy and plenty of vitamins and minerals.

Ten healthy snacks

1 A low-fat yogurt.

2 A piece of fresh fruit or a handful of dried fruit with nuts and seeds.

3   A bowl of breakfast cereal, preferably a high-fibre one with added vitamins and iron.
4   Oatcakes with some low-fat cheese.
5   Lentil and vegetable soup.
6   Wholemeal toast with yeast extract, low-fat cream cheese or mashed banana.
7   Houmous with vegetable sticks.
8   Wholemeal pitta bread filled with ham or chicken and salad.
9   A milkshake made by blending milk with a banana, strawberries, mango or peach.
10 A bowl of muesli with fruit and yogurt.

Ice cream with gherkins and other taste changes

Cravings are quite common in pregnancy, especially during the early stages. They are usually seen as quite a fun part of being pregnant. When you eat whatever it is you have been longing for, you might be surprised at just how delicious it tastes – whether it's ice cream with gherkins or something more ordinary. You might find that nothing hits the spot quite like the cream crackers you've been dreaming of all day.

The most common cravings are for fruit, sweet or salty foods, and foods with a strong flavour, such as pickles. Nobody can explain exactly why cravings occur, but it is thought that changes in hormone levels, particularly oestrogen, are partly responsible. Psychological factors also play a role. In some cultures, pregnant women do not experience cravings. Women sometimes admit that 'cravings' are a good excuse for eating things they always fancy. It's usually fine to eat the foods you crave, unless they are on the 'avoid list' or are likely to result in you gaining lots of weight.

If you have a craving for something that wouldn't usually be considered a food or drink, it is called 'pica'. Studies of pica during pregnancy have found women craving (and consuming) items such as chalk, ice, raw potato, mud, clay, coal, baby powder and laundry starch. Although most of us have heard of pregnant women eating things like this, pica appears to be more of a myth than a reality in well-fed populations – one Danish study found the incidence to be just 0.02%. However, pica appears to be more common among certain ethnic groups, including African Americans and less affluent populations around the world. Several studies have found that pica among pregnant women is associated with lower iron levels. So, if you do find yourself craving something unusual, talk to your midwife or doctor. If your iron levels haven't been tested yet, it may be a good idea to have blood tests done as soon as possible. Also, your doctor or midwife should be able to advise you about the safety or otherwise of eating particular substances.

As well as experiencing cravings, many women find they develop an aversion to particular foods or drinks during pregnancy. Even the smell of something such as wine that they enjoyed previously might make them feel nauseous. Again, hormonal changes that affect the sense of taste and smell are probably to blame. Aversions to tea, coffee, alcohol, fried or spicy food, and strong flavours and odours are all quite normal. For some women, these are the first signs of pregnancy. Aversions to certain items such as alcohol have an obvious role in protecting your baby from exposure to potentially harmful substances. However, it's not uncommon for women to develop an aversion to more healthy foods, such as meat, fish, eggs or vegetables. This sometimes happens during periods of morning sickness. You are likely to feel more normal when the sickness subsides. If you go off foods that you feel you should be eating, then it may help if someone else does the cooking or if you eat those foods cold. Then the smell isn't as strong, which can be part of the problem.

A healthy weight gain

The amount of weight women gain during pregnancy varies enormously. The extra weight isn't just the baby; it is also the placenta, amniotic fluid, increased blood volume and extra tissue in the breasts and uterus. It is also natural to lay down extra fat so that you have energy stores for breastfeeding. Some women have fluid retention during pregnancy, which contributes further to weight gain.

The general advice is that, if you eat according to your appetite, then you should gain a healthy amount of weight. Unfortunately, many women these days aren't used to eating in response to hunger and fullness. This is especially true of those who have been yo-yo dieters or have been particularly weight-conscious in the past. As a result, they can become very worried about putting on weight and may try to restrict their weight gain. Other women take the opposite view and see pregnancy as a time to relax their usual rules about avoiding fattening foods and instead eat whatever they fancy. Neither approach is good, as gaining too little or too much weight can cause health problems.

Not enough

There is a very strong association between weight gain during pregnancy and birth weight. The more weight you put on, the bigger your baby is likely to be. This might make you think that you should limit your weight gain, as a smaller baby will mean an easier birth. However, low-birth-weight babies are more likely to have health problems at birth, developmental delays as they grow up and an increased risk of heart disease in later life. In addition, girls who are small at birth have been found to be more likely to have children with raised blood pressure. So, restricting your weight gain now could have health implications for your future grandchildren.

Too much

Gaining a very large amount of weight can also have health implications for your baby. You should try not to put on more than about 12 kg (2 stone) in total, according to the Food Standards Agency. Gaining a lot of weight makes you more likely to develop high blood pressure and gestational diabetes. It also increases the chances of you having a very large baby, which can increase the risks during delivery, including the likelihood of needing a Caesarean. In addition, it increases your own risk of obesity in the future, which in turn means that you are more likely to develop heart disease, diabetes and cancer. Losing weight after having a baby isn't as easy as many people think. A Swedish study found that women who gained more than 16 kg (2.5 stone) during pregnancy were still 5.5 kg (12 lb) heavier a year after their baby was born.

You may be worried about putting on too much weight, but try not to let it become an obsession. Don't let yourself go completely but, equally, don't diet, even if you are overweight. Dieting during pregnancy is associated with an increased risk of neural tube defects and other complications.

You may know that you're putting on weight but feel happier if you don't weigh yourself at all. And in fact there isn't really any need to do so. The important thing is to try to make a conscious effort to eat as healthily as possible. You can still have occasional treats as well of course. But if you are constantly tempted by high-fat and high-sugar foods such as crisps or chocolate, then make sure you always have healthier options available (see Ten healthy snacks, page 9). Also, try eating more low-GI (glycaemic index) foods, such as lentils and oats, to stabilise your blood sugar levels and keep you feeling fuller for longer. The aim of healthy eating is to get the right combination of nutrients while getting enough, but not too many, calories.

Low-carb eating
Low-carb diets, such as the Atkins diet, could be dangerous during pregnancy. Not only can weight loss increase risks, but also the balance of nutrients is associated with a number of potential problems.

Keeping carbohydrate intake to a minimum (no bread, pasta, potatoes, etc.) means that protein foods make up a larger proportion of the diet than is usual or healthy. In animal studies, high-protein diets have been shown to increase the risk of miscarriage and genetic abnormalities. Studies in Scotland have also shown that adults whose mother had a high protein intake during pregnancy were more susceptible to raised blood pressure, insulin deficiency and heart disease in later life.

How much weight should you gain?

The amount of weight you should gain during pregnancy depends on your weight before you became pregnant. Women who are overweight need to gain much less weight than those who are underweight for optimal fetal growth. The Institute of Medicine in the USA recommends different weight gains according to pre-pregnancy body mass index (BMI), which indicates whether weight is appropriate for height. To find your pre-pregnancy BMI, either use the online calculator at http://www.eatwell.gov.uk/healthydiet/healthyweight/bmi calculator/?lang=en or follow the steps in the box below.

Calculating your BMI

By working out your BMI, you can see whether you are a healthy weight for your height.

1 Measure your height in metres. To convert from feet and inches, multiply your height in inches by 0.0254. For example, if you are 5ft 2in, this is 62 inches (12 inches to a foot), so the calculation is 62 x 0.0254 = 1.57m.

2 Measure your weight in kilograms. To convert from stones and pounds, multiply your weight in pounds by 0.454. For example, if you weigh 10 stone, this is 140lb (14lb to a stone), so the calculation is 140 x 0.454 = 63.6kg.

3 Divide your weight by your height squared. For example:

$$\frac{63.6}{1.57 \times 1.57} = 25.8$$

For a simpler idea of whether you are the right weight for your height, use the graph below. First find your height up the side and then your weight along the top or bottom, depending on whether you work in kilograms or stones and pounds.

You can then use the guidelines in the table opposite, which were calculated using data on weight gain and pregnancy outcome from thousands of women. Weight gains within the recommended ranges are associated with the lowest risk of complications during pregnancy and labour, and with the best chances of having a baby with a healthy birth weight.

Height/weight chart

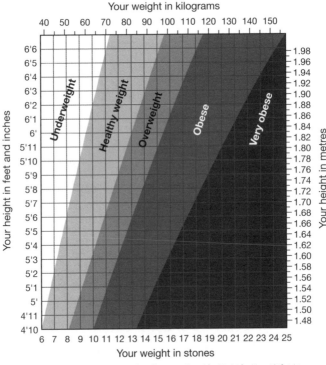

Source: Adapted from the Food Standards Agency, http://www.eatwell.gov.uk/healthydiet/healthyweight/height weightchart/ (last accessed 1 May 2008). © Crown copyright.

BMI before pregnancy	Recommended weight gain
Less than 19.8	12.5–18kg (2st–2st 12lb)
19.8–26	11.5–16kg (1st 11lb–2st 7lb)
26–29	7–11.5kg (1st –1st 11lb)
More than 29	Around 6kg (13lb)

Source: Institute of Medicine (1990) *Nutrition During Pregnancy*, Table 1.1. Washington, DC: National Academies Press. Reprinted with permission from the National Academies Press, Copyright 1990, National Academy of Sciences.

Staying active

It is important to stay active to feel healthy and maintain a general sense of well-being. Walking, swimming and yoga are all ideal forms of exercise while pregnant. They can help you feel healthier and more relaxed, so you sleep better. By keeping fit, you are likely to have more stamina for labour and an easier birth. Keeping in good shape will also help you recover more quickly after the birth and make you feel more energetic and better able to look after your baby.

Twins and more!

If you are expecting twins, triplets or even more babies, you are likely to gain more weight than a woman expecting just one. This is due not only to the weight of an extra baby but also to an extra placenta and more amniotic fluid. You are quite likely to feel particularly hungry in early pregnancy and gain more weight in the first few months.

Unfortunately, morning sickness also tends to be worse in multiple pregnancies, as circulating levels of hormones are higher in early pregnancy. Heartburn is more common too, as the uterus is larger and therefore pushes on the stomach more. There are no official guidelines regarding additional energy and calorie requirements for multiple pregnancies. However, extra calories are needed, and these should come from nutrient-rich foods. These will supply extra vitamins and minerals, including iron and vitamin A, which are more likely to be lacking in multiple pregnancies.

Foods to kick-start labour – or not

If your due date comes and goes, and nothing seems to be happening, it can be very frustrating, particularly if friends and family start phoning to see how it all went. There are many myths and old wives' tales about what you can do to kick-start labour – some more pleasant than others. With food, there are several suggestions:

- raspberry leaf tea
- pineapple
- curry.

Unfortunately, none of these actually appear to be effective. Raspberry leaf tea may help during labour (see page 105), but there is no evidence that it gets labour started. Fresh pineapple could theoretically help, as it contains an enzyme called bromelain; however, you would need to eat between seven and ten whole pineapples to get enough to have any possible effect (see page 102).

The final strategy, eating curry, has the greatest potential for getting things moving, but only if it is so hot that it causes you considerable discomfort and acts as a strong laxative. Then it could have the same effect as a dose of castor oil, which has been used for centuries to kick-start labour. It is thought that when the gut is stimulated, it in turn stimulates the uterus to cramp or spasm, thereby bringing on labour. Castor oil contains ricinoleic acid, or ricinic acid, which irritates the small intestine and has a strong laxative effect. One American study found that after a 60-ml dose, 58% of women started labour within 24 hours, compared with just 4% of untreated women. However, this was only a small study, and self-treatment is not recommended. Castor oil can result in severe nausea and cramps, persistent diarrhoea, dehydration and other complications. If you want to try castor oil or an extremely hot curry, it is important to talk to a doctor or midwife first. They will be able to advise you according to your medical history (e.g. irritable bowel syndrome or piles), the position of your baby and the condition of your cervix.

There are other non-food strategies that might help, which are less likely to have the unpleasant side effects of curry or castor oil. You could try nipple stimulation or having sex – although both these methods are thought to help only if labour is about to happen in the next few days anyway. Or you could try an alternative therapy such as homeopathy or acupuncture.

2 Foods and drinks to avoid in pregnancy

When you are pregnant, you should avoid certain foods and drinks, and cut down on others. Some, such as raw eggs, pâté and blue cheese, can lead to food poisoning. Others, including liver products, certain fish and alcohol, contain substances that could be toxic in high doses to your developing baby. As mentioned previously, you should try to avoid eating too many sugary and fatty foods such as take-aways, fizzy drinks, crisps, biscuits and sweets, which contribute to weight gain without providing essential nutrients.

This chapter gives you a complete checklist of what to avoid and what to cut down on. It then looks at particular food hazards to help explain why there are quite so many rules. This should also show that there are still plenty of tasty dishes you can eat, and that many foods can be made safe simply by taking a few extra precautions, such as thorough cooking. To find out more about the risks associated with particular foods, such as tuna, mayonnaise and goats' cheese, you can also look them up in the A–Z section (see Chapter 7).

What to avoid

The following all pose a risk to you or your baby:

- Blue-veined cheeses, such as Stilton, and soft mould-ripened cheeses, such as Brie and Camembert. These can contain listeria (see page 23).

- Raw or partially cooked eggs. Any dishes containing egg should be cooked until the yolk and white are solid. Foods such as homemade mayonnaise and mousse should be avoided.

- Unpasteurised milk, including goats' and sheep's milk, and products such as yogurt and cream made from these.

- Liver, liver products and any supplements containing high levels of vitamin A, such as cod liver oil.

- Raw or undercooked meat, including cured meats and salami. The main concern with such foods is toxoplasmosis, but they may also contain other types of food poisoning bacteria.

- Shark, swordfish and marlin. This is to avoid ingestion of mercury, which could harm the unborn baby's developing nervous system.

- Raw shellfish such as oysters, and cold dishes containing shellfish such as prawn, unless freshly prepared.

- Pâté, including vegetable pâté, to avoid the risk of listeria.

- Alcohol. Drinking it during pregnancy increases the risk of miscarriage and birth defects.

What to cut down on

There are certain foods and drinks that you don't need to avoid completely but should consume only in moderation:

- Tuna should be limited to no more than two fresh steaks or four cans per week, as it contains small traces of mercury.

- You shouldn't have more than two portions of oily fish per week, to avoid consuming harmful levels of pollutants.

- Caffeine intake should be limited to no more than 300 mg per day, which is equivalent to about two to three mugs of instant coffee or two cups of real coffee.

Peanuts

Peanuts are a special case, as most women can safely eat them during pregnancy. However, the Food Standards Agency recommends that pregnant women avoid eating peanuts if they have a family history of allergies, including asthma, eczema or hay fever (see pages xvi and 101).

Beware! Food hygiene hazards

During pregnancy, you are more susceptible to food poisoning. This is because your immune system undergoes certain changes to prevent your body reacting against your growing baby. To avoid getting food poisoning, it is important to pay special attention to food hygiene.

Most forms of food poisoning are caused by bacteria. There is usually a delay between eating the contaminated food and the development of any symptoms. This is known as the incubation period and it can range from a few hours to several days, depending on the bacteria's method of attack. Some bacteria stick to the lining of the intestine and destroy cells directly. These cause symptoms such as nausea, vomiting, abdominal cramps and diarrhoea. Others produce a toxin that is absorbed and can produce symptoms elsewhere, such as headache. In warm environments, bacteria multiply rapidly, for example at picnics and barbeques and on buffet tables. In such environments, a single bacterium can become several million bacteria within eight hours.

You can reduce your risks of getting food poisoning considerably by taking some sensible precautions when you are preparing and storing food, and when you eat out or get a take-away.

Preparing food

- Always wash your hands before eating or preparing food.
- Wash all fruit and vegetables before eating, including bags of salad leaves labelled as 'washed and ready to eat'.
- Keep your kitchen clean and don't allow pets on tables and kitchen work surfaces.
- Before eating hot foods, make sure they are piping hot right the way through. This is particularly important for ready meals, pies and processed meat products such as burgers and sausages.
- When using a microwave, follow the instructions carefully, including stirring and standing times. Then check the food is cooked all the way through before eating.
- After handling raw eggs, meat and poultry, wash your hands and any utensils thoroughly with hot soapy water. Kitchen worktops should be washed well after any spills or splashes from these foods. If you don't wash and dry your hands thoroughly, bacteria can easily be spread to fridge handles, cutlery and other foods.

Storing food

- Make sure the temperature of your fridge is below 5°C and your freezer below –18°C.
- Check the use-by date and storage instructions on packaging, and stick to them.

- Store any raw meat at the bottom of the fridge, wrapped and separate from food that is ready to eat. Raw eggs should also be stored carefully.

- Cool and refrigerate any leftovers within an hour of cooking and eat them within 24 hours.

Take-aways and eating out

When someone else is preparing your food, it is impossible to be 100% sure about hygiene standards. It is best to eat only in places you trust, and it is generally safer to choose hot dishes rather than cold ones such as salads. If you get a take-away meal and it's not piping hot when it arrives, you could heat it in the microwave as an extra precaution.

Don't be afraid to ask about ingredients or information about how dishes have been cooked, for example whether the mayonnaise is homemade or whether the ice cream contains raw eggs. Most places will be happy to help, and a bit of embarrassment now is better than worrying about something later.

Different types of food poisoning

Listeria

Listeria (*Listeria monocytogenes*) is a type of bacteria found in some foods, soil, vegetation and sewage. It can cause an illness called listeriosis, which can have serious consequences during pregnancy. It is impossible to tell whether a food is contaminated with listeria, as it will look, smell and taste normal. Listeria is found in small amounts in many foods, but some, such as pâté, may have much higher levels.

Pregnant women are about 20 times more likely than other adults to get listeriosis, because of hormonal changes affecting their immune system. Although the illness is unlikely to be serious for the mother, it can result in miscarriage, premature delivery, stillbirth or severe illness in newborn babies.

Cases of food poisoning from listeria have increased in recent years. Between 20 and 25 cases of listeriosis are reported in pregnant women in the UK each year, according to the Health Protection Agency (HPA). It is still fairly rare, but if you are pregnant, there are certain precautions you can take to reduce your risk of infection. It is important to follow the general food hygiene rules for storing and preparing foods, but there are also certain foods that are more likely to contain listeria and are best avoided completely during pregnancy:

- Blue-veined cheeses and soft mould-ripened cheeses (for a full list, see page 79).
- Pâté, including liver pâté and vegetable pâté (see page 100).
- Unpasteurised dairy products, including milk, cream, yogurt and ice cream.
- Pre-packaged salad leaves – these need to be re-washed thoroughly.
- Ready meals such as lasagne and curry – the manufacturer's re-heating guidelines should be followed carefully, and you should also check that the food is piping hot all the way through.

Symptoms of listeriosis can take up to two or three months to appear after exposure and may include fever, a mild flu-like illness or diarrhoea. These symptoms can, of course, have other causes. If you are concerned, it is best to see your GP, who may ask for blood or urine tests. If you do have listeriosis, it can usually be treated successfully with antibiotics.

Toxoplasmosis

This is an infection caused by a microscopic parasite called *Toxoplasma gondii*, which is found in meat, soil and cat faeces. More than half of people with toxoplasmosis don't know they have it, but in others it can cause flu-like symptoms or more severe symptoms similar to those of glandular fever. If a woman becomes infected during pregnancy or in the two to three months before conception, it can cause miscarriage, stillbirth or a range of birth defects, including hydrocephalus and brain lesions.

The most common cause of toxoplasmosis is consumption of raw or undercooked meat, so you should only eat meat that has been thoroughly cooked and shows no traces of blood or pinkness. Raw cured meats such as Parma ham should also be avoided. Other causes of toxoplasmosis include unpasteurised milk products and any food contaminated with soil. As well as making sure that fruit and vegetables are completely free of soil, women are advised to wear gloves when gardening and handling cat litter, and to wash their hands carefully afterwards.

If you think you may have toxoplasmosis, it is important to see your doctor. You can have blood tests; if these are positive, then your baby can also be tested via amniocentesis or cordocentesis. Infection is not always passed from a mother to her baby, and prompt antibiotic treatment can prevent the baby from becoming infected.

Salmonella

This is one of the commonest causes of food poisoning. It differs from the listeria and toxoplasmosis bugs because it doesn't cross the placenta to the baby. However, salmonella can make you very ill, with a high temperature that could harm your unborn child. Symptoms include heavy vomiting and diarrhoea, but the effects vary. There are 200 strains of salmonella. High-risk foods include raw and partially cooked eggs (including those in dishes such as home-made mayonnaise and ice cream) and poultry and meat that hasn't been cooked well.

Brucella

This bacteria is sometimes found in unpasteurised milk and dairy products, including cheese and yogurt. Infection can result in fever, illness and miscarriage. It is rare in the UK but more common in Middle Eastern countries and some Mediterranean countries, including Spain. If you are travelling abroad it is best to ensure that any dairy products are made from pasteurised milk. At home, avoid 'country' or 'locally made' cheeses from these countries.

E. coli

Most strains of *Escherichia coli* (*E. coli*) bacteria are harmless, but some can cause severe food poisoning. These produce verocytoxins and are known as verocytoxin-producing *E. coli* (VTECs). In the UK E0157 is the most common VTEC, but in other countries E0111 and E026 are more common.

The foods most likely to contain harmful strains of *E. coli* are undercooked minced beef (e.g. in burgers) and unpasteurised milk. *E. coli* can also be transmitted directly from infected animals, people and soil. If a pregnant woman contracts *E. coli*, it isn't transmitted to the fetus. However, symptoms can be serious and include bloody diarrhoea and abdominal cramps. The illness can also have serious complications, such as severe anaemia and problems of the nervous system and kidneys.

Mercury
This metal can have a toxic effect on the development of an unborn or very young baby's nervous system. The FSA recommends that pregnant women avoid eating shark, swordfish and marlin, as these fish have been found to contain high levels of mercury. Lower levels of mercury have been found in tuna, so consumption of this fish should be limited to no more than two fresh tuna steaks or four medium cans a week.

Alcohol

The Department of Health advises pregnant women and those trying to get pregnant not to drink any alcohol. Avoiding alcohol during the first three months of pregnancy is particularly important, according to NICE. However, if you do choose to drink, you should not have more than 1 to 2 units of alcohol once or twice a week at any stage of pregnancy, and you shouldn't get drunk. At this low level of consumption, there is no evidence of harm.

			Units of alcohol
Wine	175-ml glass if 12% ABV		2
	250-ml glass if 12% ABV		3
	250-ml glass if 14%		3.5
Beer	275-ml bottle of beer or $\frac{1}{2}$ pint (5% ABV), e.g. Heineken®, Becks®, Carlsberg Export®		1.5
	330-ml bottle of Sol® (4.5%)		1.5
	440-ml can of 4% lager, e.g. Carling®, Carlsberg®, Fosters®		2
Alcopops (per 275-ml bottle)	Archer's Aqua Peach®		1.5
	Bacardi Breezer®		1.5
	Smirnoff Ice®		1.5
	WKD Vodka Blue®		1.5
Spirits e.g. Smirnoff Red®, Bacardi® are 37.5%	Single	(25 ml)	1
		(35 ml)	1.3
	Double	(50 ml)	2
		(70 ml)	2.6
	Tequila (50-ml shot)		2

Remember the advice refers to 1 or 2 units, not 1 or 2 drinks.

ABV is % alcohol by volume.

A high alcohol intake can reduce your fertility and ability to con-ceive. It also affects the absorption of some nutrients and may in-crease the risk of miscarriage in the early stages of pregnancy, possibly before you know you are pregnant.

Heavy alcohol consumption during pregnancy (more than 10 units a week) is associated with fetal alcohol syndrome (FAS). FAS is characterised by low birth weight and length, a variety of congenital abnormalities and facial malformations. In recent years, several studies have suggested that moderate alcohol consumption (around 4 units per week) may adversely affect the neurological development of some fetuses.

The term fetal alcohol syndrome disorder (FASD) is now used to describe a whole range of problems, including FAS and also less severe conditions. It is estimated that in Britain, more than 6000 children each year, or 1 in every 100 babies, is affected. The effects range from learning difficulties to facial abnormalities, limb damage and heart defects. There are different risks associated with drinking at different stages of pregnancy. The effects of drinking alcohol appear to be more severe in some women, particularly if they have a poor diet and a low intake of certain vitamins, including B vitamins.

Some experts disagree with the government advice, saying there is no evidence to support a complete ban on alcohol. The problem is that it is not clear-cut. Any observational survey has to rely on women's own reports about how much they have been drinking, which may not be reliable for many reasons. Also, women who choose to drink may have a different lifestyle from those who don't. They may be more likely to smoke or less likely to take supplements, and there is no way of distinguishing which aspect of their behaviour is affecting the health and development of their babies.

The only way to settle the question once and for all would be a study in which different groups of women consumed specific amounts of alcohol throughout pregnancy. It would then be possible to see at what level of alcohol the incidence of birth defects and developmental problems increased. Of course, this would be completely unethical. Experts have to give advice based on the limited evidence available. As it is known that alcohol passes through the placenta, and there is no proven safe level of exposure for a fetus, most agree that caution is the best option. The only way to ensure that your baby is not affected by alcohol is to stop drinking completely.

Caffeine

Caffeine is found in tea, coffee, cola, chocolate, energy drinks such as Red Bull, and some medication such as cold and flu remedies, headache treatments and diuretics. It is a stimulant and diuretic (it makes you wee).

It is fine to have up to 300 mg of caffeine per day during pregnancy, according to the FSA. This is equivalent to about two cups of coffee and a bar of chocolate. Having more than this can increase the risk of having a low-birth-weight baby or even a miscarriage. Caffeine crosses the placenta and affects your baby in the same way it affects you.

One, much publicised study carried out in the USA found that women consuming more than 200 mg of caffeine a day had twice the miscarriage risk of those consuming no caffeine. Even those with lower caffeine intakes were at increased risk of miscarriage compared with the abstainers. On the basis of this evidence, some experts now believe that it is best to avoid caffeine completely during the first 12 weeks of pregnancy, when the risk of miscarriage is highest. After that, levels below 200 mg are thought to be safe. The advice of the FSA remains the same (up to 300 mg is safe); however, the FSA is looking at all the evidence, including the American research and new data on the caffeine intake of 2500 women in the UK, and it may change its advice in the future.

To help stay within the limit, use the table overleaf as a guide.

		Caffeine content (mg)
Chocolate	Plain (50-g bar)	Up to 50
	Milk (50-g bar)	25
	Drinking chocolate (cup)	1–8
Coffee	Filter or percolator (cup)	100–115
	Instant (cup)	75
	Instant (mug)	100
	Espresso (single)	75–100
	Cappuccino/latte (regular)	150–200
	Americano (regular)	225
	Decaffeinated (cup)	4
Cola	Regular or diet (330-ml can)	40
Energy drink	Containing caffeine or guarana (can)	Up to 80
Tea	Medium strength (cup)	50

The amount of caffeine varies with the blend of tealeaves or coffee beans, the strength of tea or coffee, and the serving size.

3 The who's who of nutrients – what you *should* eat

We all know that nutrients are important, but what exactly are they? Basically nutrients are any substances found in food or drink that are essential to health. There are two types. **Macronutrients** – protein, carbohydrate and fat – provide energy (calories) and have specific roles in maintaining health. **Micronutrients –** vitamins and minerals (e.g. iron and calcium) – are equally important but are needed in smaller amounts.

Here we look at each nutrient in turn, giving a brief run-down on what it's for, how much you need and where to find it. However, if you want a shortcut to good meals that contain all these nutrients in the right amount, go to page 48, where you'll find some sample meal planners.

Protein

What it's for: Protein provides amino acids, one of the basic building blocks of human tissue. Protein is needed for the growth of the fetus and placenta and for changes in the mother's body that occur during pregnancy. In addition, protein is needed for the production of breast milk.

Amount needed: When you are pregnant or breastfeeding, you need about 51g of protein a day. This is just 6g more than is needed before pregnancy. In practice, there is usually no need to increase your protein intake during pregnancy, since the average (non-pregnant) women consumes about 60g of protein a day anyway.

Where it's found: Good sources of protein include lean meat, chicken and fish (21–28g per 100g), eggs (14g in two eggs), milk (10g per half-pint/300ml) and other dairy products such as yogurt (7g per small pot). Non-animal sources of protein include baked beans (11g in half a tin), chickpeas and kidney beans (7g per 100g), tofu (7–10g per 100g) and cereal products such as bread (7g per two slices). Vegetable sources of protein generally contain fewer essential amino acids, but anyone eating a mixed diet should get all the amino acids they need.

Carbohydrates

What they're for: Carbohydrates are the main source of energy in our diets. They contain fewer calories per gram than fat, making carbohydrate-rich foods better than fatty ones for avoiding excess weight gain. Low carbohydrate diets can negatively affect a baby's long-term health, including increasing the risk of high blood pressure (see page 12).

Amount needed: There are no specific guidelines as to how much carbohydrate you should eat each day – it depends on how many calories you need. However, it is estimated that about 50% of a person's calories should come from carbohydrates.

Where they're found: Carbohydrates come in the form of either sugars or starch. Sugars are found in many foods, including fruit and milk, where they are accompanied by essential nutrients such as vitamin C and calcium. They are also found in products such as cakes and sweets, but these contain few or no useful nutrients, so you should limit your intake of them. Among starchy foods, unrefined are better than refined varieties. That means choosing foods such as wholemeal bread, brown rice and pasta, and wholegrain breakfast cereals such as branflakes, rather than white bread, white rice and cornflakes. Wholegrain products provide extra fibre and more vitamins and minerals than refined (usually white) foods.

Low-GI carbs

The glycaemic index, or GI, of a carbohydrate-rich food ('carb') measures its impact on blood sugar or blood glucose levels. Low-GI foods, such as oats and lentils, are broken down slowly, so they keep you feeling full for longer and produce only a small fluctuation in blood glucose. High-GI foods, by contrast, result in blood sugar levels increasing more rapidly and to a higher level, and dropping off more steeply. High-GI foods include white bread, cakes, biscuits and sugary drinks.

One study found that consuming low-GI foods as part of a healthy (but not low-calorie) diet was good for pregnancy. It reduced the risk of having a baby with neural tube defects, particularly among overweight women. Another study found that women consuming more low-GI foods were less likely to gain a large amount of weight or have a baby that was very large for its gestational age.

Although substituting high-GI for lower-GI foods offers several advantages, typical low-GI diets aimed at weight loss are not appropriate for pregnancy (see page 12). If you want to find the GI of particular foods, there are a variety of guides available, and some food products now include a GI rating on the label.

Fibre

What it's for: There are two types of dietary fibre. Insoluble fibre, generally known as roughage, helps food move through the digestive system so you don't get constipated. Soluble fibre, found in oats and lentils, helps to stabilise blood sugar levels.

Amount needed: Adults should consume about 18g of fibre (technically known as non-starch polysaccharides, or NSP) per day. This should come from foods that contain fibre naturally, such as wholegrains, fruit and vegetables, rather than fibre drinks or bran sprinkled on other foods (see page 76).

Where it's found: High-fibre (NSP) foods include breakfast cereals such as branflakes (5g per 40g bowl) and wholemeal bread (4.5g per two slices). Vegetables, including peas (4g per portion) and carrots (2g per portion), are another good source. Fresh fruit such as apples and oranges (1.5–2g per fruit) and dried fruit such as raisins (1g per 50g portion) are further alternatives.

Fats

What they're for: Fats get a bad press, but some fatty acids (the building blocks for fat) are essential for good health. There are three different types of fatty acid, which are found in varying amounts in foods. These are:

- **Saturated** – the type found in meat and dairy products such as cheese. These are not essential, and a high intake increases the risk of heart disease.
- **Monounsaturated** – found in olive oil and rapeseed oil, and also not essential to health.

- **Polyunsaturated** – some polyunsaturated fatty acids (PUFAs) are known as 'essential fatty acids'. They can't be produced by the body and must be supplied by the diet. There are two families of essential fatty acids:

  — **Omega 6** (n-6) – derived from linoleic acid (LA) and found in vegetable oils such as sunflower oil.

  — **Omega 3** (n-3) – derived from alpha linolenic acid (ALA) and found in some vegetable oils such as rapeseed and flaxseed oils. Longer-chain omega 3s, docosahexaenoic acid (DHA) and eicosapentaenoic acid (EPA), are found in oily fish and some fortified foods and supplements. They are not generally considered essential for adults, as they can be made from ALA, but many experts believe that they are beneficial during pregnancy and in early infancy for brain and eye development. It is estimated that during pregnancy a baby accumulates at least 10 g of DHA, and 6–7 g of this is during the last trimester, mainly for brain development.

As well as providing essential fatty acids, fat is needed in the diet for absorption of the fat-soluble vitamins A, D, E and K.

Amount needed: Fat shouldn't make up more than 35% of your calorie intake. However, it is estimated that about 30 g of fat is needed each day for the absorption of adequate amounts of fat-soluble vitamins. For pregnant and breastfeeding women, it is also estimated that at least 200 mg of DHA is required per day, according to a group of over 30 experts set up by the European Commission. The advice from the Perinatal Lipid Metabolism (PeriLip) research group and the Early Nutrition Programming project was based on their 2007 review of the evidence relating to omega 3 fatty acids and fetal and infant development. Other expert groups believe that recommendations should be set higher, at 300 mg per day for optimal fetal development.

Where they're found: Obvious sources of fat are cooking oils, which are almost 100% fat, and spreads such as butter and margarine

(12g fat per tablespoon). Fat is also found in dairy produce such as cheese (10g per 30-g portion of Cheddar) and in cheesy foods such as pizza (up to 36g in a 200-g portion). Other high-fat foods include pastry products (e.g. 27g per 75-g sausage roll), cakes (26g per 100-g sponge cake) and chocolate (15g per 50-g bar).

The best dietary sources of DHA are oily fish, such as salmon and mackerel (800–1500mg per portion). See page 97 for advice about oily fish consumption.

The main sources of ALA are flaxseeds (3.8g per tablespoon of ground seeds), flaxseed oil (8g per tablespoon), rapeseed oil (1.6g per tablespoon) and walnuts (2.5g per 25-g handful).

The body can convert ALA (found in flaxseeds) to the beneficial long-chain omega 3s DHA and EPA (found in oily fish), but not very efficiently. You are unlikely to get enough long-chain omega 3s by eating ALA-rich foods alone. Part of the problem is that the conversion of ALA to DHA is disrupted by high intakes of LA (an n-6 fat found in many foods). This is because the same enzymes are used for metabolising LA as for ALA. Reducing the ratio of LA to ALA (n-6 to n-3) fatty acids in the diet can help. In practice, this can be achieved by replacing sunflower oil or corn oil with rapeseed oil, flaxseed oil or olive oil and eating more ALA-rich foods.

Metabolising ALA to longer-chain EPA and DHA can also be limited by a lack of certain micronutrients, including iron, calcium, zinc and vitamin B_{12}. There is speculation that conversion of ALA to DHA is boosted during pregnancy, but this has not been proven. A study of pregnant Dutch women who were given ALA (via a fortified margarine) found no increase in the mothers' or babies' levels of DHA at birth compared with a control group. A similar study in the USA in which breastfeeding mothers were given 20g of flaxseed oil daily found no change in their DHA levels or in the DHA levels in their breast milk. The researchers in both studies conclude that the most efficient way of meeting an infant's DHA requirement is to increase the mother's intake of pre-formed DHA. So, if you don't eat oily fish and foods fortified with long-chain omega 3s, you might like to consider taking a supplement containing DHA – either a fish oil supplement or one made from algae oils (see page 53).

Omega 3s – what's all the fuss?

Research has shown that a good intake of long-chain omega 3s during pregnancy reduces the risk of having a low-birth-weight or premature baby. A Danish study of nearly 8000 pregnant women found low birth weight and premature birth were three times more common for mothers who did not eat any fish compared with those who had the highest intakes (just under two portions a week). Although this is a fairly high intake, the researchers noted that risks were reduced significantly for women consuming even small amounts of fish (less than one portion a week).

As well as having a positive influence on the outcome of pregnancy, your DHA intake is also important for your child's development. Consuming higher levels of DHA during pregnancy and after birth has been found to have beneficial effects on a baby's visual acuity, cognitive function, attention, maturity of sleep patterns and spontaneous motor activity. A high intake may also reduce a baby's sensitivity to common allergy triggers, including egg, and reduce the severity of eczema if it occurs.

Vitamins and minerals

There are two types of vitamins: water soluble and fat soluble. The water-soluble vitamins are the B vitamins and vitamin C. The fat-soluble vitamins are vitamins A, D and E. Water-soluble vitamins are easily lost if foods containing them are overcooked or boiled in lots of water that is then thrown away. Water-soluble vitamins are also lost more easily from the body. If you have a large intake of water-soluble vitamins, much of them will be lost in the urine. In contrast, if you have a large intake of fat-soluble vitamins, there is a greater potential for problems, as your body has to work harder to deal with them. A high vitamin A intake can be dangerous, and pregnant women are advised to avoid certain foods to reduce the risk of excess intake. Likewise, taking iron supplements during pregnancy isn't advisable, unless blood tests have shown that you have low iron levels (see page 53). You are extremely unlikely to have an excessively high intake of any vitamin or mineral (other than vitamin A) from diet alone. A pregnancy-specific multivitamin and mineral supplement should also in general contain only the amount of nutrients you might find in foods. However, the effect of taking supplements containing large doses of vitamins or mineral is unknown, and excess intakes are possible.

Vitamin A

What it's for: This vitamin is needed for a strong immune system and the development of healthy skin and eyes. One of the first signs of deficiency is night blindness (an inability to see in dim light), but more severe deficiency can result in permanent eye damage. It is also important for the development and maturation of your baby's lungs.

Amount needed: During pregnancy you need 700 µg of vitamin A (retinol equivalents) per day. This increases to 950 µg per day while breastfeeding.

Where it's found: There are two forms of vitamin A: retinol and beta-carotene. Retinol is found in animal sources, including liver (13 000–40 000 µg per 100 g), liver pâté (7330 µg per 100 g), milk (58 µg per half-pint) and eggs (110 µg each). Beta-carotene is found in vegetables, particularly orange-coloured varieties such as carrots (1000 µg per portion[1]), mango (240 µg per portion[1]), cantaloupe melon (133 µg per portion[1]) and apricots (54 µg per portion[1]).

High intakes: Although you need some vitamin A, if you have a very high intake, levels in your body can build up. As it is a fat-soluble vitamin, excess amounts aren't eliminated through the urine.

[1] 1ug of beta-carotene is equivalent to approximately 6µg of retinol. The vitamin A content of foods containing beta-carotene is given here as retinol equivalents. They don't contain any retinol, but this allows direct comparison with the level of vitamin A recommended.

Vitamin A in the form of retinol is teratogenic. This means that a high intake (more than about 3300 µg per day) is associated with an increase in birth defects. For this reason, pregnant women and women trying for a baby are advised not to eat liver or liver products. They should also avoid supplements containing vitamin A, such as cod liver oil, unless advised by their doctor to take them. It is perfectly safe to consume other foods containing retinol, such as milk and cheese, as these have much lower levels. You can also eat foods containing high levels of beta-carotene during pregnancy; the worst effect this could have is to make your skin look slightly orange. Some experts believe that women need to increase their intake of beta-carotene during pregnancy, as vitamin A deficiency can be a real risk, particularly for women having twins and those having babies close together.

Folic acid

What it's for: It reduces the risk (by as much as 70%) of your baby developing a neural tube defect, such as spina bifida, if taken from before conception until week 12 of pregnancy. It also reduces the risk of cleft palate and harelip, and it works with vitamin B_{12} to form healthy red blood cells.

Amount needed: Before pregnancy you need 200 µg of folic acid a day. This increases to 300 µg a day during pregnancy and 260 µg a day if you are breastfeeding. You should also take folic acid supplements before pregnancy and in the first 12 weeks. This is recommended even if you have a good diet, as it is almost impossible to get enough folic acid, in a form that is easily absorbed, from food alone.

Where it's found: Folic acid is found naturally as folate in food. It is one of the B vitamins. Good sources are broccoli (65 µg per 85-g portion), oranges (50 µg each), fortified breakfast cereal (33–100 µg per bowl), peas (40 µg per two tablespoons), yeast extract such as Marmite (25–100 µg per portion) and milk (15 µg per 250-ml glass).

Folic acid is easily destroyed by cooking, so it's important not to overcook vegetables.

See page 52 for information on folic acid supplements.

Vitamin B$_2$ (riboflavin)

What it's for: You need this vitamin for the conversion of fats, protein and carbohydrates into energy. Deficiency results in cracked skin at the corners of the mouth and skin problems around the nose, eyes and tongue.

Amount needed: You need 1.4 mg per day during pregnancy and 1.6 mg per day while breastfeeding. If you consume too much, it will be excreted in your urine.

Where it's found: It is found in a variety of foods, particularly those of animal origin such as milk (0.5 mg per half pint) and cheese (0.1 mg per 25 g). It is also found in wholegrain cereals such as branflakes (0.5 mg per bowl), mushrooms (0.3 mg per portion), almonds (0.2 mg per 20-g portion) and yeast extract (0.3 mg per 4 g).

Vitamin B$_6$ (pyridoxine)

What it's for: Needed for the metabolism of protein and release of energy from foods. Vitamin B$_6$ is also needed for the development of a healthy nervous system and red blood cells. Deficiency is rare, but there is some evidence that women with low levels are less likely to become pregnant and more likely to miscarry in early pregnancy.

Amount needed: You need about 1.2 mg per day. There is no extra requirement for pregnancy or breastfeeding.

Where it's found: The best sources are fish such as salmon (1.2 mg per portion) and tuna (0.6 mg per tin), nuts (0.2 mg per 30-g handful of hazelnuts, peanuts or walnuts), bananas (0.3–0.5 mg per banana, depending on size) and some vegetables (avocados, red peppers and potatoes provide about 0.3mg per 100g).

See page 54 for information on vitamin B_6 supplements.

Vitamin B_{12}

What it's for: This vitamin is important for healthy red blood cells, the release of energy from food, and the development and normal functioning of the nervous system. It is also needed for the body to be able to process folic acid. Pregnant women with low vitamin B_{12} levels appear to be at slightly greater risk of having a baby with spina bifida. However, the evidence for this is only limited, compared with the very strong evidence of an association between folic acid and spina bifida prevention.

Amount needed: During pregnancy 1.5μg per day is needed. This increases to 2.0μg per day while breastfeeding.

Where it's found: Vitamin B_{12} is found in almost all foods of animal origin, including beef, pork and lamb (about 2μg per 100g), salmon (8.4μg per portion), tuna (5.4μg per tin), milk (1.1μg per half-pint), yogurt (0.3μg per pot) and eggs (1.0μg each). It isn't found naturally in foods of plant origin, so vegetarians tend to have a lower intake. However, yeast extract is a rich source (0.3μg per teaspoonful) and many breakfast cereals and soya products are fortified with vitamin B_{12}.

Choline

This is not by strict definition a vitamin, although it is sometimes grouped with the B vitamins. Choline is important for lipid metabolism and for the transmission of nerve impulses. There is also some evidence that choline plays a role in memory. The main sources of choline are milk, eggs and liver, but it is also found in meat and fish at lower levels. The body can make small amounts of

▶

choline, but not enough for optimal health. Individual requirements appear to vary and be dependent on genetic makeup. It is thought that additional choline is required during pregnancy, but a varied diet should supply adequate amounts.

Vitamin C (ascorbic acid)

What it's for: This vitamin protects cells and keeps them healthy. Vitamin C is particularly important for wound healing. It also increases the absorption of iron from foods of plant origin such as breakfast cereals, bread, beans and vegetables (see page 45).

Amount needed: During pregnancy, 50 mg is needed per day. This increases to 70 mg per day while breastfeeding.

Where it's found: Fruits such as oranges (54 mg each) and strawberries (62 mg per portion), potatoes (10 mg per 100 g) and many vegetables, including broccoli (50 mg per portion) and cauliflower (28 mg per portion). Vitamin C is easily lost, so it is best to steam or lightly cook vegetables. If fruit is cut, it should be eaten as soon as possible.

Vitamin D

What it's for: This vitamin helps with absorption of calcium and builds strong healthy bones. It is particularly important during the later stages of pregnancy. If you don't get enough vitamin D during pregnancy or while breastfeeding, your baby may have low vitamin D and calcium levels. This can lead to the baby developing seizures in the first months of life. It also puts the baby at risk of developing the bone disease rickets, which results in a softening of the bones as they grow and is characterised by bowed legs. Other symptoms of deficiency in babies are poor teeth formation and general ill health. Poor vitamin D status during pregnancy is also associated with reduced bone mass in childhood and may increase the risk of osteoporosis in later life.

Amount needed: Most adults can get enough vitamin D from normal exposure to the sun. Ultraviolet B (UVB) radiation converts a vitamin D precursor in the skin to the active form of the vitamin. People with darker skins are at greater risk of deficiency, as they require longer exposure to sunlight to make the same amount of vitamin D. Women who have limited exposure to sunlight are also at greater risk of deficiency, for example women who remain covered for religious reasons when they go outside, and shift workers. Women who are pregnant or breastfeeding require extra vitamin D and are advised to take a supplement containing 10 µg vitamin D each day. If you're on a low income, you may be eligible for free supplements through the Healthy Start scheme (see page 57).

Supplements are particularly important in the winter months when there may not be enough sunlight of the appropriate wavelength to stimulate the production of sufficient vitamin D. During the summer months it is estimated that 15 minutes of sunlight on the arms, shoulders and head each day will supply enough vitamin D. During the winter months, people living at latitudes above 52 degrees (in the UK, people living north of Birmingham) are thought to receive no UV light of the appropriate wavelength to make vitamin D in their skin.

Where it's found: Very few foods contain vitamin D naturally. Good sources include oily fish such as sardines (6.4 µg per tin), salmon (3.5–7 µg per portion) and eggs (1 µg each). There are also several foods that are fortified with vitamin D, including all margarines (0.8 µg per 10 g) and many breakfast cereals (0.6–3.0 µg per bowl).

Vitamin E

What it's for: Vitamin E is an antioxidant and helps protect cells, particularly those of the nervous system, from damage. There is some evidence to suggest that eating a diet high in vitamin E during pregnancy may protect your baby against developing asthma and other allergies in later life.

Amount needed: Requirements for vitamin E depend on the amount of polyunsaturated fatty acids (PUFA) you consume. Individuals with higher PUFA intakes require more vitamin E, so there are no recommended levels for the population. However, intakes around 4–5mg per day appear to be satisfactory for women who are pregnant or breastfeeding.

Where it's found: Vitamin E is found in most fruit and vegetables, including spinach (1.4mg per portion), broccoli (1mg per portion), carrots (0.5mg per portion), tomatoes (1mg each) and apples (0.6mg each). It is also found in nuts such as almonds and hazelnuts (7mg per 30g) and in seed oils, for example rapeseed oil (3mg per tablespoon) and sunflower oil (7mg per tablespoon).

Calcium

What it's for: Calcium helps build strong bones and teeth. It also regulates muscle contraction and is needed for normal blood clotting.

Amount needed: Before and during pregnancy you need 700mg per day. For breastfeeding, this increases to 1250mg per day. To help your body absorb calcium, it's important to have enough vitamin D. You need to be especially careful about getting enough calcium if you are a vegan, or a teenager, or if you don't drink much milk or eat many dairy products.

Where it's found: Milk (350mg per half-pint), yogurt (225mg per pot), cheese (200mg per 30-g portion), fish eaten with soft bones, such as canned sardines (275mg per half-tin), cabbage and broccoli (35mg per portion) and bread (40mg per slice). Some food products are also fortified with calcium, including some soya milks and desserts and some orange juice.

Iron

What it's for: Iron is needed for healthy red blood cells, which carry oxygen around the body. During pregnancy, iron requirements are increased not only to supply the baby and placenta but also to produce extra red blood cells for your own circulation. Most pregnant women are routinely monitored in case they are deficient in iron or anaemic. If your iron levels are low, you may feel especially tired and lethargic or even faint. It can also affect your baby–iron-deficiency anaemia is associated with lower birth weight and prematurity. In addition, evidence is emerging to suggest that a good iron intake during pregnancy may reduce the risk of your child developing asthma.

Amount needed: 14.8 mg of iron is required per day.

Where it's found: Good sources of iron include meat and fish. The darker the meat is, the higher the iron content tends to be. For example, beef (2 mg per 100 g) contains more iron than chicken (1.2 mg per 100 g) or trout (1.4 mg per portion). Iron is also found in dried fruits such as apricots and raisins (1 mg per handful), baked beans (3 mg per half-tin) and wholemeal bread (1 mg per slice). Many breakfast cereals also have iron added to them (3–8 mg per bowl), and this is an important source for many women. Some foods thought to be good sources of iron are not as useful as commonly believed, including spinach (page 111) and Guinness (page 90).

See page 53 for information on iron supplements.

Easy ways to boost iron absorption
The iron in meat and fish is absorbed more easily than that in foods of plant origin. However, you can boost the amount of iron your body absorbs from food such as cereals, bread and lentils by having vitamin C at the same time. You could have strawberries with breakfast cereal, fruit salad after a sandwich, or a glass of orange juice with beans on toast. It also helps if you avoid tea or coffee at

▶

meal times and for about an hour afterwards, as they contain polyphenols, which bind to iron, making it more difficult to absorb. One study found that orange juice increased iron absorption by 85% whereas tea reduced iron absorption by 62%.

Zinc

What it's for: Zinc is needed to make new cells and enzymes and to help with wound healing. The body also needs zinc to process the protein, carbohydrates and fats we eat.

Amount needed: During pregnancy you need 7 mg of zinc per day. While breastfeeding, this increases to 13 mg per day for the first four months and 9.5 mg a day thereafter.

Where it's found: Good sources of zinc include chicken (2.0 mg per 100 g), beef (4.6 mg per 100 g) and other meat, milk (1.1 mg per half-pint) and other dairy products such as cheese (0.7 mg per 30 g of Cheddar). Zinc is also found in cereal products, particularly whole-grain varieties such as branflakes (1 mg per bowl) and wholemeal bread (1.4 mg in two slices).

Iodine

What it's for: Iodine is important for the development of the nervous system, particularly during the first three months of pregnancy. Babies of iodine-deficient women can have mental retardation. Iodine is also needed for the production of thyroid hormones. Deficiency is extremely rare in European countries, but women with marginal intakes can start to show signs of deficiency during pregnancy. The most obvious sign of deficiency is goitre, which is a large swelling on the neck.

Amount needed: 140 µg per day.

Where it's found: The best source of iodine is fish (70–420μg per portion), but milk (43μg per half-pint) and other dairy products such as cheese (13μg per 30g of Cheddar) are also important. Cereals and other foods of plant origin such as beans and vegetables contain very little iodine, so vegans tend to have an extremely low intake unless they consume seaweed or foods fortified with iodine.

Selenium

What it's for: Selenium is an antioxidant and therefore protects against cell damage. Selenium also plays an important role in the immune system, thyroid hormone metabolism and reproduction. Research suggests that having a good intake of selenium during pregnancy may reduce the risk of your baby developing eczema and wheezing (an early warning sign for asthma).

Amount needed: Women are advised to consume 60μg of selenium per day during pregnancy and 75μg per day while breastfeeding.

Where it's found: Good sources of selenium include Brazil nuts (300 μg per 20-g portion), tuna (117μg per tin), lentils (40μg per 100g), white fish such as cod (47μg per portion) and bread (25μg in two slices).

Fluoride

What it's for: Fluoride is needed for strong tooth enamel and bone formation.

Amount needed: In the UK, there are no recommendations for daily intake of fluoride.

Where it's found: Tea is the main source of fluoride in the UK. It is also found in water, milk and fish that are eaten with bones, such as sardines.

See page 55 for information on fluoride supplements.

From nutrients to meals – sample meal plans

Learning about the key nutrients for pregnancy can be helpful, but for you to really benefit this information has to be translated into everyday eating. Below is a one-week meal planner to show you how you can get all the nutrients you need from meals and snacks. This isn't a menu plan for you to follow, but it should give you an idea of what a healthy balanced diet really looks like.

DAY 1
Breakfast   Porridge and a handful of dried apricots.
Lunch   Tomato and lentil soup with a wholemeal roll,
             and a peach.
Dinner   Grilled salmon, a baked potato with cottage cheese,
             and some broccoli and carrots. Apple crumble and
             dairy vanilla ice cream.
Snacks   Oatcakes with cream cheese and grapes.

DAY 2
Breakfast   Branflakes with a sliced banana.
Lunch   A tuna and sweetcorn sandwich with salad, and a
             cranberry juice.
Dinner   Chickpea and sweet potato curry with chapatti.
             Fresh raspberries with natural yogurt.
Snacks   Mixed nut flapjack and an apple.

DAY 3
Breakfast   Muesli.
Lunch   Baked beans on wholemeal toast, and a glass
              of orange juice. Fresh fruit salad.
Dinner   Stir-fried chicken with peppers, mange tout, baby
              corn, carrots and egg noodles.
Snacks   A slice of carrot cake and fresh strawberry
              milkshake.

DAY 4
Breakfast   A grapefruit, and wholemeal toast with Marmite.
Lunch   Cheese and tomato toasted sandwich with
              watercress and pine nut salad.
Dinner   Pasta with roast vegetables (e.g. peppers,
              tomatoes and courgette), and a pot of yogurt.
Snacks   A banana. Houmous with carrot sticks and pitta
              bread.

DAY 5
Breakfast   Scrambled eggs on granary toast with grilled
              tomatoes.
Lunch   Mixed bean salad with tomatoes and avocado, and a
              slice of rye bread. Pot of yogurt.
Dinner   Roast lamb with potatoes, broccoli, red cabbage
              and carrots. Glass of sparkling grape juice. Rice
              pudding.
Snacks   An apple and a bag of dried fruit and seeds.

DAY 6
Breakfast   Weetabix with mixed berries.
Lunch   Slice of vegetarian pizza and an orange.
Dinner   Fish pie with peas.
Snacks   Date and walnut cookie and a smoothie.

The who's who of nutrients – what you *should* eat   **49**

DAY 7

Breakfast	Muesli and orange juice.
Lunch	Leek and potato soup with bread and cream cheese. A pear.
Dinner	Chinese beef with mixed peppers, stir-fried cabbage and rice.
Snacks	Bowl of cereal and banana. Slice of chocolate cheesecake.

4 Supplements – who needs what and why

For most people in good health, a well-balanced diet provides all the necessary nutrients. However, during pregnancy, there is clear evidence that certain supplements are beneficial. Supplements containing folic acid and vitamin D are recommended for all pregnant women, irrespective of how well or how badly they eat. Other supplements, such as iron tablets, should be taken during pregnancy only if blood tests show they are needed. Then there are multivitamin and mineral supplements and omega 3 capsules. The manufacturers would have you believe that every mum-to-be needs them, but it's important to think about your own diet and to look at the evidence before deciding whether they are really for you.

The FSA advises all pregnant women to take:

- 400 µg of folic acid daily for the first 12 weeks of pregnancy;
- 10 µg of vitamin D daily for the entire course of pregnancy.

Folic acid supplements

There is strong evidence that folic acid supplements reduce the risk of having a baby with a neural tube defect (NTD) such as spina bifida or anencephaly. In fact, trials with folic acid supplements had to be stopped early because the benefits were so clear that it was unethical to continue giving some women a placebo.

Ideally you should start taking folic acid supplements before you become pregnant, but otherwise begin as soon as possible and continue until week 12 of pregnancy. It's safe to continue taking folic acid beyond 12 weeks, but there is generally no need if you are eating well. Supplements are available from chemists and most supermarkets quite cheaply, or you may be eligible for free supplements (see page 57).

Supplements containing 400 μg (sometimes written as 0.4 mg, 400 mcg or 400 micrograms) of folic acid are recommended for most women. However, some women may benefit from even higher doses of up to 5 mg (5000 μg). If you have had a previous pregnancy affected by a NTD, or if you or your partner has a family history of NTDs, or if you have diabetes, then ask your doctor whether you need to take a higher dose of folic acid. Unless you have been advised to take more than the recommended 400 μg per day, it is best not to take more than 1000 μg (1 mg) per day.

Vitamin D supplements

The FSA advises women to take supplements containing 10 μg (10 mcg) of vitamin D throughout pregnancy and while breastfeeding. This is needed for the absorption of calcium and to build strong bones. Low levels of vitamin D during pregnancy can be detrimental to both mother and baby and can result in weak bones and infantile seizures (see page 42).

About a third of young women have low levels of vitamin D in their blood. Those most at risk are women who don't get much sunlight, women of South Asian, African, Caribbean or Middle Eastern descent, women who are obese, and women who have recently been pregnant. Women with low levels of vitamin D don't have adequate stores to draw on when they become pregnant and, as you are unlikely to know whether you are among the one in three with low levels, supplements are a good idea.

Iron supplements

You need to take iron supplements during pregnancy only if blood tests show that you have low levels of iron, in which case your midwife or doctor will prescribe them. If your iron levels are normal, then it may actually be harmful to take high doses of iron (i.e. more than is found in pregnancy multivitamin and mineral preparations).

Some women find that the iron supplements they are prescribed (usually ferrous sulphate) cause unpleasant side effects, including nausea and constipation. If so, it may help to take the supplement with food. If this doesn't work, you may find it worth switching to a different iron supplement, such as Spatone. Any iron supplements you are prescribed while you are pregnant will be free, but you'll probably have to pay for alternatives – but if it makes you feel better, it's generally worth it. To increase the amount of iron you absorb from supplements, drink orange juice at the same time as taking the supplement and avoid having tea or coffee for an hour after taking them.

Omega 3 supplements

There are several different types of omega 3 supplement available. Some contain ALA, which is one of the shorter-chain omega 3s found in various seed oils, including flaxseed. ALA can be converted to the beneficial long-chain omega 3 fatty acids DHA and EPA, but only to a limited extent. It is better to take supplements containing readymade DHA (see page 36).

Supplements containing long-chain omega 3s (including DHA and EPA) are derived either from oily fish or from algal sources, which are suitable for vegetarians. Guidelines suggest taking between 200 mg and 300 mg of DHA per day, but fish oil supplements containing up to 1g (1000 mg) of DHA per day or 2.7 g of long-chain omega 3s per day have been used in research studies without any adverse effects (apart from belching and a nasty taste). There has not been much research on DHA supplements made from algae. However, the studies that have been done, in non-pregnant individuals, suggest that they are effective in raising blood DHA levels and that they appear to be safe and well tolerated.

Supplements containing cod liver oil, or other fish liver oils, are also high in beneficial omega 3s. However, they are not suitable for pregnancy because they contain high levels of vitamin A, which could be harmful to your baby.

Vitamin B$_6$ supplements

There is a small amount of evidence suggesting that taking vitamin B$_6$ supplements can relieve nausea and vomiting during pregnancy in some women. However, the FSA advises against taking more than 10 mg of supplemental vitamin B$_6$ a day. Taking large doses (200 mg a day) is associated with nerve damage and loss of feeling in the hands and feet, which may be irreversible. Taking a smaller dose, around 100 mg a day for a short period, may be quite safe, but nobody really knows. If you want to try supplements, it is best to talk to your doctor before starting.

Research in Thailand found that vitamin B$_6$ supplements weren't as effective as either ginger or acupressure at relieving nausea and vomiting, so you may like to get some wristbands and ginger before following this route.

Fluoride supplements

These are not recommended. There is some evidence that taking fluoride supplements during pregnancy reduces the risk of your child developing tooth decay. However, this research is controversial, as other studies have found no benefit. There is also some suggestion, although it has not been researched properly, that taking fluoride supplements in pregnancy could adversely affect fetal brain development.

Multivitamin and mineral supplements

If, for any reason, you think your nutrient intake is inadequate, then you may want to take a multivitamin and mineral supplement. A general supplement for pregnancy and breastfeeding provides a good safeguard for women with limited diets, for example vegetarian women and women who don't eat dairy foods. Some others, such as diabetic women and teenagers, may also benefit. If you are concerned, ask for further advice from your doctor or midwife, or ask to be referred to a dietician.

The safest supplements are those available on the high street labelled as suitable for pregnancy and breastfeeding. It is not advisable to take a multivitamin and mineral supplement that is not specifically formulated for pregnancy, as it may not contain the right balance of nutrients; for example, it may have too much vitamin A or not enough folic acid or vitamin D for pregnancy. It is not a good idea to take high doses of specific nutrients either, as some have unknown effects. A study with high doses of vitamins C and E found that the desired effect of preventing pre-eclampsia wasn't achieved but that there were an increased number of babies with low birth weight (weighing less than 2.5 kg).

For a healthy woman with a mixed diet (including meat, fish, dairy produce, fruit and vegetables) the benefits of taking a multi-vitamin and mineral supplement during pregnancy are unclear. Some research shows that taking a supplement before pregnancy may reduce the risk of premature delivery (before 37 weeks of pregnancy) and taking a supplement during pregnancy may decrease the risk of birth defects (e.g. neural tube defects and urinary tract defects), childhood leukaemia and brain tumours. However, one study found that multivitamin supplements were actually associated with an increased risk of multiple congenital anomalies. On balance, the evidence suggests that they either are beneficial or have no effect.

It is difficult to determine the impact of supplements, because women who take them are less likely to smoke or drink alcohol and more likely to eat well and exercise compared with women who don't take supplements. It could be that any reported health benefits are the result of these factors rather than of the supplements themselves.

If you do decide to take a supplement, remember that it is not a substitute for a good diet. For one thing, real foods such as fruit and vegetables contain many beneficial phytochemicals, such as lycopene in tomatoes and anthocyanins in blackberries and aubergines, which are not found in most supplements. A good diet is also high in fibre and low in salt and contains the right balance of fatty acids. So, if you take a supplement, you should still try to eat as well as possible. It is best to take any supplements during or after a meal in order to maximise nutrient absorption.

Diabetic mums and supplements

If you have diabetes, it may be a good idea for you to take a general pregnancy multivitamin supplement. A study conducted in the USA found that although diabetic women had an increased risk of having a baby with a birth defect such as hydrocephaly, a heart defect or cleft palate, those who took a multivitamin supplement before and during pregnancy had no greater risk than non-diabetic women.

Healthy Start

If you are on a low income, you may be eligible for free supplements through the Healthy Start scheme. This scheme helps pregnant women and mothers of young children who are on a low income or receiving certain benefits. In addition, all pregnant women under the age of 18 qualify. Women who are eligible receive free vitamin supplements (containing folic acid and vitamins C and D) and vouchers for free fruit, vegetables and milk. Women who aren't eligible for free Healthy Start supplements can buy them from community pharmacies. To find out more about Healthy Start, see Resources and useful contacts (page 144) or ask your doctor, midwife or health visitor for details.

5 Common complaints and how to deal with them

It would be great if every woman could spend her pregnancy feeling radiant with health and vitality. However, few of us make it through the whole nine months without at least a bit of queasiness or constipation. Some women feel downright rotten for some or even most of their pregnancy, and the majority fall somewhere in between. But there are things you can do to make yourself feel better. If you have morning sickness or any form of digestive problem, fairly simple dietary changes can make a big difference.

Conditions generally considered more serious – gestational diabetes and pre-eclampsia – are covered at the end of the chapter. These may not immediately seem diet-related but, as you'll see, nutrition can play a role.

Morning sickness

Despite its name, 'morning sickness' can occur at any time of the day. Some women find that it gets worse if they are feeling tired, stressed or hungry. It can also be triggered by certain odours, such as cooking smells or strong aftershave.

The majority of women experience some feelings of nausea during pregnancy, although some suffer much more than others. Symptoms tend to be worst at around nine to ten weeks and disappear by about the fourteenth week. The exact cause of morning sickness isn't known, but it is thought to be related to the sudden rise in blood levels of a hormone called human chorionic gonadotropin (hCG) in early pregnancy. You may worry that your baby is suffering too. However, sickness is actually a sign that your hormones are changing as they should. Even if you are not able to eat much, your baby is very unlikely to be affected (see page xiii).

There is no single treatment that works for all women, but different strategies can be helpful. You could try the following:

- Eat little and often. By eating small, carbohydrate-rich meals or snacks every couple of hours, you can stop your blood sugar levels dropping too low, which can make you feel worse.

- Eat some dry crackers or biscuits in bed before getting up in the morning.

- Avoid foods that you find trigger nausea, such as fatty or spicy dishes or foods with a strong odour. It may be better to eat certain foods cold or, if you can, get someone else to do the cooking.

- Avoid other triggers. Some women find that the smell of petrol or perfume is a problem or that travelling in the back seat of a car makes them feel worse.

- Vitamin B_6 supplements may help (see page 54).

- Have plenty of fluids, but avoid caffeine and alcohol, to prevent dehydration.

- Have ginger in any form, for example ginger tea or ginger biscuits (see page 89).

- Get more fresh air.

- Rest and sleep as much as possible.

- Get some seasickness wristbands from a chemist. These act on the acupressure point for nausea. Some trials, though not all, have found that they are effective for morning sickness.

- Sip cider vinegar in water (see page 81).
- Complementary therapies such as aromatherapy, homeopathy and acupuncture work for some women.

A very small number of women suffer from severe vomiting during pregnancy (hyperemesis gravidarum), which can lead to dehydration and weight loss. If you are severely affected and can't even keep water down, see your doctor.

Heartburn

Whereas morning sickness is most common at the beginning of pregnancy, heartburn is more likely to be a problem in the last three months. The main symptom is a burning sensation in the chest, caused by acids going back up the food pipe from the stomach. A muscle valve usually prevents this from happening, but during pregnancy it becomes more relaxed because of hormonal changes.

Heartburn can be particularly bad after a large meal or during activities that involve bending over, such as cleaning the floor or even just picking something up. The pressure of the baby on the stomach can make heartburn even worse towards the end of pregnancy. However, the symptoms may lessen when the baby's head becomes engaged: as it moves further down into the pelvis ready for birth, the pressure on the stomach is reduced. The good news is that when the baby is delivered, heartburn usually disappears almost instantly.

There are several things you can do to ease the symptoms of heartburn:

- Wear loose-fitting clothes to reduce extra pressure on your stomach.
- Avoid becoming too full, by eating little and often instead of having large meals. Also, don't drink too much at mealtimes.

- Try to identify trigger foods and avoid them, especially in the evening. Common culprits include spicy food, citrus fruits, rich and fatty foods, tea and coffee, and bananas.
- When you eat, sit upright instead of slouching and try not to rush.
- Try to stay sitting upright for a while after meals. When you go to bed, prop yourself up with several pillows.
- Milk is good for neutralising the acid and easing symptoms, so try drinking a small glass before bed or have some ready to sip during the night.
- Homeopathy, aromatherapy and yoga may all help.
- If symptoms are severe, talk to your midwife or doctor. They will probably prescribe a suitable anti-reflux medicine.

Constipation

Constipation is more common than usual during pregnancy because of hormonal changes. Increasing progesterone levels cause all the muscles in your body, including intestinal muscles, to relax, so food moves through your intestines more slowly. This helps your body to absorb more nutrients from the food you eat, but it can also lead to constipation. In addition, the pressure of your baby on your bowels can make going to the toilet more difficult. Iron tablets can also cause constipation (see page 53).

To treat constipation, try the following:

- Eat plenty of fibre-rich foods (e.g. wholemeal bread, wholegrain breakfast cereal) and lots of fruit and vegetables.
- Have some prunes or prune juice (see page 104).
- Drink plenty of water, but avoid having too much caffeine, as it can contribute to dehydration, which makes constipation worse.
- Take some gentle exercise, such as walking, swimming or yoga.

- When you go to the toilet, relax and take your time.
- Switch iron supplements if necessary.

If this doesn't help, talk to your midwife or doctor; they may pre-scribe laxatives that are safe to take during pregnancy. Not all lax-atives are safe in pregnancy.

Wind and bloating

As well as constipation, pregnant women often have more wind, bloating and general digestive discomfort than normal. Because food spends longer in the large intestine (see above), it has more time to ferment and produce more gas or wind.

To relieve the symptoms of wind and bloating, try the following:

- Avoid foods that are particular triggers. Different foods seem to affect different people, but beans, cabbage and onions are common culprits. To prevent your diet becoming too limited, you may occasionally want to have individual trigger foods, but avoid having several at the same time.
- Don't eat large meals.
- Try to relax and sit up tall at mealtimes.
- When you eat, chew properly and avoid gulping air, by eating slowly and not talking too much.
- Avoid swallowing air when you drink by using a cup or glass rather than a bottle or straw.
- Take gentle exercise such as yoga or walking to help keep your digestive system working efficiently.
- Avoid fizzy drinks.

If you are feeling pain rather than just discomfort, talk to your doc-tor or midwife as soon as possible.

Haemorrhoids (piles)

Piles or haemorrhoids are varicose veins around the rectum and anus (back passage). They may develop for the first time during pregnancy, or existing piles may get worse. Piles are exacerbated by straining when you go to the toilet and by constipation. The best way to prevent piles from developing, and to treat them if you get them, is to follow the advice for dealing with constipation. You should also try not to strain on the toilet. If the piles are very inflamed and itchy, talk to your midwife or doctor about a suitable cream to ease your discomfort.

Sometimes piles become worse after the birth – particularly if it is a difficult vaginal delivery. However, the good news is that as you recover from the birth, piles become much less of a problem.

Diarrhoea

Although constipation is a much more common complaint than diarrhoea during pregnancy, some women do find that diarrhoea is a problem. This is nothing to worry about unless the diarrhoea is severe and continues for more than a few days. If this is the case, you should see your GP or midwife for further tests, such as a stool culture, to rule out salmonella and other infections.

Like so many pregnancy problems, diarrhoea can be caused by changing hormone levels. It is not a problem in itself, but it can cause dehydration. If you have diarrhoea, it is important to drink plenty of water or take rehydration powder available from a pharmacy. Taking a probiotic yogurt or drink may also help.

If you find that diarrhoea is a problem towards the end of pregnancy, it can be one of the signs that labour is imminent.

Restless legs

Restless leg syndrome (RLS) involves a strong urge to move the legs and also sometimes the arms. Women generally find symptoms are worse when they settle down for a much-needed rest, particularly at night. RLS can occur at any stage of life, but it is two to three times more likely during pregnancy, particularly in the last trimester. Typically symptoms disappear after the baby is born.

It is not clear what causes RLS, but people with the syndrome have been found to have lower levels of dopamine in a region of the brain known as the substantia niagra. Iron is known to be important in the production of dopamine, and low iron levels may be part of the problem. Certainly RLS appears to be more common in pregnant women with low iron levels, and symptoms tend to reduce when iron supplements are given. In addition, folic acid supplements have been found to help alleviate symptoms, although the reason for this is less clear.

Gestational diabetes

This is a temporary form of diabetes that occurs during pregnancy. It develops when hormones from the placenta interfere with insulin, the hormone that regulates blood sugar levels. As a result, the levels of glucose or sugar in your blood can rise and dip steeply. Gestational diabetes is more common in women with a family history of diabetes, in women who have had a very large baby before, and in older mums. During pregnancy, urine samples are tested routinely for glucose, as this is usually the first sign of a problem. A single positive urine test is not usually a cause for concern, but if traces of glucose are found on several occasions you may be sent for further tests.

Gestational diabetes is usually detected at 24–28 weeks of pregnancy. Women who develop the condition, like those who have diabetes before pregnancy, are likely to have bigger-than-average babies. This in turn increases the likelihood of problems during delivery. However, if the condition is controlled carefully, it should not harm you or your baby.

It is important that blood sugar levels are kept as stable as possible, so that the baby doesn't receive extra glucose. This can usually be achieved with a change in diet, but sometimes it requires insulin. Avoiding high-sugar foods and drinks and consuming low-GI carbohydrates is an important part of the dietary management of diabetes. If you have gestational diabetes, you will receive appropriate advice from your midwife, doctor or a dietician. After the baby is born, the condition usually goes away completely.

Pre-eclampsia

This is a serious pregnancy disorder characterised by high blood pressure and protein in the urine. Other symptoms may include headaches, blurred vision and swelling. You are more likely to develop the condition if you are overweight, aged over 35 or expecting more than one baby, or if any of your close relatives has had it. Untreated, it can progress to eclampsia, which results in fitting and, very occasionally, death. However, drugs can usually be given to treat the symptoms and, when necessary, the baby will be delivered early.

Diet appears to play a role in reducing the risk of developing pre-eclampsia. The condition seems to be more common in women with a low intake of antioxidants. Having a healthy diet (including foods rich in vitamin C and vitamin E) is particularly important for women at increased risk. Research has been carried out to see whether taking antioxidant supplements containing vitamins C and E helps in prevention as well; however, these trials, rather surprisingly, found that pre-eclampsia was just as common when supplements were taken. In addition, women taking the supplements were more likely to have a low-birth-weight baby. Further research is being carried out, but because of these unwanted results supplements containing large doses of vitamins C and E are no longer recommended. Pregnancy multivitamin supplements usually contain lower doses of these vitamins and shouldn't be a problem. In fact, another research trial found that pregnancy multivitamins might help in preventing pre-eclampsia. The effect of calcium supplements has also been investigated; these supplements may help women who are deficient in calcium, but they are unlikely to work for others. Garlic may help too, by lowering blood pressure, but research is inconclusive.

6 A healthy vegetarian pregnancy

Vegetarians sometimes come under pressure to start eating meat during pregnancy 'for the good of the baby'. But there really is no need. Babies born to vegetarians are usually just as big and healthy as those born to non-vegetarians. It is perfectly possible to have a healthy diet for pregnancy without eating meat or fish. You just need to avoid the possible pitfalls. So you can reassure any well-meaning relatives and friends that there's no need for you to tuck into that steak any time soon.

In some ways, vegetarian diets are positively beneficial. They tend to be lower in saturated fat and higher in fibre, beta-carotene, folic acid, vitamins C and E and magnesium. However, they usually contain lower levels of some key nutrients too, such as protein, omega 3 fatty acids, vitamin B_{12} and zinc. When you know the potential problems, it is fairly simple to make sure you don't miss out on anything important. With a little bit of planning, you can make sure your vegetarian diet is as good as, if not better than, that of any meat eater. Even if you are not a strict vegetarian but one of the growing number of women who eat very little meat, you need to think about the same dietary issues. You should also find the same advice helpful.

One of the most basic nutrient requirements is for protein, and vegetarians tend to get less of it than meat eaters. However, protein intake can vary widely. People who live on vegetables and cereals tend to have lower intakes of protein, but vegetarians who eat dairy foods and eggs along with a variety of soya products, pulses, seeds and nuts have much more. Vegetable sources of protein are sometimes described as being of low biological value because they contain fewer essential amino acids. However, you can get all the essential amino acids you need by eating a mixture of different cereals, peas, beans, lentils, seeds and nuts. If you eat dairy foods and eggs too, then there is really no need to worry. If you don't tend to eat these different foods regularly, then it is a good idea to start trying to include a source of protein in every meal.

Vegetarians have also been found to have very low intakes of long-chain omega 3 fatty acids, as these are found mainly in oily fish. You can increase your intake by eating Columbus eggs (see page 82) and food products fortified with long-chain omega 3s (DHA and EPA) from algal sources. Consuming foods such as flaxseed, flaxseed oil and walnuts will increase your intake of alpha linolenic acid ALA, a short-chain omega 3. However, ALA needs to be converted to the beneficial long-chain omega 3s, and that conversion is limited (see page 36). It is higher in women than men, but ALA is still unlikely to provide optimal levels of DHA. Another problem is that vegetarians tend to have higher than average intakes of omega 6 fatty acids, including linoleic acid (LA), which inhibit the conversion of ALA to the long-chain omega 3s.

To improve the fatty acid content of your diet and to optimise the amount of long-chain omega 3s that your body produces, it is a good idea to switch from sunflower oil or corn oil or margarine (which have high levels of LA) to soya bean or rapeseed oil. You may also like to take an omega 3 supplement (see page 53). The Vegetarian Society suggests that pregnant and breastfeeding women should consider boosting their diet with a direct source of DHA, such as a supplement derived from algae in a non-gelatine capsule.

When it comes to vitamins and minerals, a lack of iron is the most likely problem for vegetarians. You have a greater risk of becoming anaemic, but you can improve your iron levels by eating more foods fortified with iron and taking steps to increase the amount of iron you actually absorb. This includes having a glass of orange juice with meals, avoiding tea and coffee at mealtimes, and making sure not every meal is high in fibre. Having a very high fibre intake can also restrict your absorption of zinc and calcium, so the odd low-fibre meal or snack is a good idea.

Not getting enough calcium is sometimes highlighted as a potential problem for vegetarians, but this is really an issue only if you don't have much milk or dairy products in your diet. If that is the case, you should think about alternative sources of calcium (see Extra advice for vegans, below). Vegetarians who eat plenty of dairy foods are likely to have a calcium intake similar to the average non-vegetarian's.

Vitamin B_{12} is another one to watch. Again, women who eat few dairy foods and women who don't eat eggs are most at risk of missing out. There are plenty of alternative sources of vitamin B_{12}, but you must check food labels to find them. Foods of plant origin don't naturally contain this vitamin, so you need to find those that are fortified. Most breakfast cereals have added vitamin B_{12}, but not muesli or any organic cereals. Many vegetarian dairy alternatives, such as rice milk and soya puddings, are also fortified with calcium and vitamin B_{12}, but reading the labels is the only way to find out which.

There has been some concern in recent years over high intakes of soya in pregnancy. Vegetarian mothers were found to be more likely than meat eaters to have babies with hypospadius (see page 110). However, evidence from countries with a high intake of soya suggests that normal soya consumption is fine.

On a more positive note, vegetarians have been found to have higher levels of folic acid during pregnancy, because they eat more fruit and vegetables. But this doesn't mean that folic acid supplements aren't needed – these are recommended for all women, however high their folate intake. Vegetarians also have slightly higher intakes of magnesium than meat eaters and, possibly related to this, a lower incidence of leg cramps in the last trimester of pregnancy.

Your diet will generally be much better if you include a variety of different beans, pulses, lentils, seeds and nuts, as well as yeast extract and other fortified foods. The Vegetarian Society (see Resources and useful contacts, page 145) provides a useful information sheet for pregnancy, including a guide to the number of portions from different food groups required each day. If you are still unsure about the adequacy of your diet, it might be a good idea to take a pregnancy multivitamin and mineral supplement to be on the safe side.

Meat cravings

Cravings for meat are fairly rare among pregnant vegetarians, although you'll probably be asked about them. Vegetarians tend to have similar cravings to other women, although they are more likely to crave pickles and salty or savoury foods such as yeast extract, and less likely to crave fruit and sweet foods.

Extra advice for vegans

Vegans, who consume only foods of plant origin, need to be aware of a few extra issues. Your diet can still be perfectly adequate while you are pregnant or breastfeeding, but you need to plan a bit more carefully and you are more likely to benefit from supplements. Vegans, just like vegetarians, tend to have lower intakes of protein, vitamin B_{12} and omega 3 fatty acids, and they are more likely to have low iron levels. The advice for vegetarians above therefore applies to vegans too.

In addition, you need to ensure you don't miss out on the essential nutrients that vegetarians get from milk and eggs, particularly calcium, vitamin D and iodine (see page 46). If you drink soya or rice milk, make sure you choose one that is fortified with calcium and vitamins D and B_{12}. It is also a good idea to look out for other fortified foods, including orange juice with added calcium, burger mixes, breakfast cereals and puddings. A vitamin D supplement is recommended for all pregnant and breastfeeding women, but it is particularly important for vegans. You may also choose to take a general multivitamin supplement (see page 55).

7 The A–Z of foods and ingredients

In this section of the book, you can look up any food or ingredient to find out whether during pregnancy and while breastfeeding it is:

✓   Safe to eat

✘   Best avoided

✓ ✘ OK in moderation or under certain circumstances

Some items don't have a symbol because the jury is still out. For these items, all the evidence is provided so that you can make up your own mind about whether or not you want to consume them. If you eat something and then notice later that you shouldn't have, try not to worry: the risks are generally small (see page xiv).

Additives The FSA considers all additives used in the UK to be safe for consumption during pregnancy. When considering the safety of any additive, the FSA looks at the reproductive toxicity of a chemical and its ability to alter genetic material. Although the safety of individual additives is tested, there is some concern about the possible effect of consuming a combination of many different additives at the same time – the so-called 'cocktail effect'. Another concern is that foods containing lots of additives generally are overprocessed, high in fat, salt and sugar, and low in essential vitamins and minerals. Ideally you should keep foods containing additives to a minimum and instead eat plenty of unprocessed foods such as fruit, vegetables, beans and wholegrains. See also *artificial sweeteners, nitrites* and *sulphites*.

✔ **Almonds** A good source of protein, copper, niacin, riboflavin and vitamin E. There is no need to avoid almonds unless you are allergic to them.

Artificial sweeteners The most commonly used artificial sweeteners in the UK are acesulphame K (acesulphame potassium), aspartame (also known as NutraSweet®), saccharin and sucralose. The FSA considers all of these to be safe for use in pregnancy and while breastfeeding, but some people are concerned that we still don't know their real effect on pregnant women or their babies. As there is some controversy, if you consume artificial sweeteners, then it is best to do so only in moderation.

Acesulphame K is found in many diet drinks, fat-free yogurts and other reduced-calorie foods such as puddings and salad cream. Some experts believe it could cause problems during pregnancy, but there is no scientific evidence to back this up.

Aspartame is found in most diet drinks, as well as chewing gum, fat-free yogurts and some cold and flu medicines. It does not cross the placenta to the baby. A small number of scientists have raised safety concerns over aspartame, but there is no scientific evidence and experts generally consider it safe for use in pregnancy and while breastfeeding, if consumed in moderation. One group of women who do need to avoid aspartame, however, are those with the genetic disorder phenylketonuria (PKU), as they cannot metabolise it.

Saccharin is used in diet drinks, juice drinks and salad cream. It is the most controversial of the sweeteners as it has been shown to cross the placenta into the baby's bloodstream and remain there for some time. There is no clear-cut evidence, but animal experiments suggest that high consumption of saccharin during pregnancy could lead to birth defects. At very high levels, it has also been linked with bladder cancer. It is probably best avoided during pregnancy and while breastfeeding. However, if you have had some accidentally, don't worry: the risk, if any, is very low.

Sucralose is a slightly different type of sweetener, which is found in Splenda® (granulated and tablets). It is made from sugar, but it is in a form that the body can't absorb. It has not been studied extensively, but there does not appear to be any evidence that it causes harm.

Bananas A good healthy snack to have when energy levels drop ✓ when you're pregnant or breastfeeding. Some women find that bananas cause heartburn, but otherwise there's no need to avoid them.

Barbequed food Make sure all meat, burgers, sausages, fish, etc. are cooked properly, otherwise there is a risk of food poisoning. Even if something looks cooked on the outside, check that it's piping hot in the centre. Also, try to avoid heavily charred food: the cooking process produces polycyclic aromatic hydrocarbons (PAHs) and heterocyclic amines (HAs), including some carcinogenic chemicals that could be harmful during pregnancy. It is best to keep intake to a minimum, though no safe level has been established. At barbeques, it's also important to check that salads have been washed thoroughly and to steer clear of food that's been sitting outside for a long time, because food poisoning bugs multiply rapidly in warm weather.

Basil This is one of several herbs that act as a uterine stimulant ✓ when concentrated or used in very large amounts. Therefore you should avoid using basil oil (commonly used for aromatherapy) during pregnancy. However, it is safe to use basil in cooking.

✘ **Béarnaise sauce/Bernaise sauce** This usually contains partially cooked egg yolk and so should be avoided as it carries a risk of salmonella poisoning. It is possible to make Béarnaise sauce with pasteurised egg instead, in which case it is safe.

✘ **Beer** Once believed to be good for breastfeeding, but research has shown that this is a myth (see page xviii). For safety in pregnancy, see the information on alcohol on page 26.

✘ **Bran** The outer layer of cereal grains, such as wheat and rice, is called bran. It's a concentrated form of dietary fibre. Sprinkling bran on your food may help to relieve constipation, but it will also reduce the absorption of some vitamins and minerals, including iron and zinc. It is much better to eat fibre-rich foods such as wholegrain cereals (e.g. wholemeal bread, brown rice), pulses (e.g. lentils, beans) and fruit and vegetables, as these contain higher levels of essential nutrients.

✔✘ **Breakfast cereal** It's good to start the day with breakfast cereal. It also makes a healthy snack when you're pregnant or breastfeeding and feeling hungry between meals. Try to eat a cereal that's fortified with vitamins and minerals, including folic acid and iron, as these are particularly important at this time. Organic cereals are not fortified in the UK, and neither are some budget-value ranges of cereals, so check the label to find out. It is also a good idea to choose a high-fibre breakfast cereal to help prevent constipation.

✔ **Brie** Should be avoided because of the risk of listeria, which could harm your unborn baby. This includes Brie made with pasteurised or unpasteurised milk. However, dishes such as deep-fried Brie, where the cheese is piping hot, are safe, because any listeria is killed during cooking. See page 23 for more about listeria.

✘ **Caesar salad** The dressing on Caesar salad usually contains raw egg, which carries a risk of salmonella, so it is best avoided while pregnant. See page 25 for more about salmonella.

Calabash chalk This is a type of chalk (also known as Calabar stone, ✖
La Craie, Argile, Nzu and Mabele) used to alleviate morning sickness. It is traditionally used by women from West Africa and is im-
ported from Africa to the UK. However, it is not recommended, as
it has been found to contain high levels of lead, which could harm
your baby's developing nervous system.

Camembert This is a soft cheese and should be avoided during ✖
pregnancy because of the risk of listeria. This includes Camembert
made from pasteurised or unpasteurised milk. However, dishes
such as deep-fried Camembert, where the cheese is piping hot, are
safe, because any listeria will be killed during cooking. See page 23
for more about listeria.

Chalk White chalk is calcium carbonate, which the body can use
just like the calcium in food. If you experience a craving for chalk, or
anything else that isn't normally considered a food or drink, it is
known as 'pica' (see page 10). Eating small amounts of white chalk
is unlikely to do any harm. However, consuming large quantities
could cause the calcium level in your blood to become too high,
which could cause problems for you and your baby. It is not advisable to eat coloured chalk, as the colourings it contains may not be
the same as those used for food and will not have been tested to
see whether they can be safely consumed.

Cheddar cheese This is a hard cheese and is safe to eat whether ✔
made from pasteurised or unpasteurised milk.

Cheese Some cheeses should not be eaten during pregnancy as ✖
they could be contaminated with listeria. This applies to soft,
mould-ripened cheeses (e.g. Brie) and blue-veined cheeses (e.g.
Stilton), whether they are made from pasteurised or unpasteurised
milk. You should also avoid soft cheeses made from unpasteurised
goats' and sheep's milk. However, thorough cooking kills listeria, so
it should be safe to eat these cheeses if they are part of a hot dish,

e.g. on a pizza or in a sauce – you just need to make sure that they are properly cooked and piping hot all the way through.

✔ Hard cheeses (e.g. Cheddar, Edam) are safer because they are more acidic and contain less moisture, so they're less likely to allow bacteria to grow. These are considered safe whether they are made from pasteurised or unpasteurised milk.

Feta cheese and soft cheeses (e.g. mozzarella, ricotta, cottage cheese) are also safe. However, you should buy them pre-packaged and eat them before the use-by date. It is best to avoid buying them from delicatessen counters, where cross-contamination from other foods may occur.

CHEESES THAT ARE SAFE

Austrian smoked cheese
Babybel
Boursin
Caerphilly
Cheddar
Cheese spread, e.g. Dairylea, Laughing Cow, Primula
Cheestrings
Cheshire
Cottage cheese
Cream cheese, e.g. Philadelphia, or similar own-brand products
    described as 'soft cheese'
Double Gloucester
Edam
Emmental
Feta
Goats' cheese: hard goats' cheese, e.g. St Helen's Farm hard
    goats' cheese, and cheese described as full-fat or medium-fat
    goats' milk cheese, which doesn't have a rind
Gouda
Gruyere
Halloumi
Havarti

Jarlsberg
Lancashire
Leerdammer
Manchego
Mascarpone
Mozzarella
Paneer
Parmesan/Parmigiano or similar Italian hard cheese (including those
    made from unpasteurised milk)
Processed cheese
Quark
Red Leicester
Ricotta
Roullé
Wensleydale

CHEESES TO AVOID

Blue d'Auverge
Blue Shropshire
Blue Vinney
Brie
Cambozola/Cambozala/Cambozola blue Brie
Camembert
Castello blue
Castello white
Chaumes
Cornish Yarg
Crème de Saint Agur
Danish Blue
Dolcelatte
Dovedale
Goats' cheese: Chèvre, Capricorn Somerset goats' cheese, any
    goats' cheese with a rind like Brie or described as being ripened
    or mould-ripened

▶

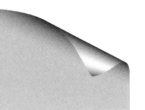

Gorgonzola/blue Gorgonzola
Pont L'eveque or Demi Pont L'eveque
Roquefort
Saint Agur
Stilton

NB The rules for organic cheese are the same as those for non-organic cheese, for both cheeses that are safe and cheeses to avoid.

✓ **Cheesecake** It is fine to eat cheesecake that has been cooked, sometimes described as a baked cheesecake. You can also safely eat cheesecake sold in supermarkets and similar shops, as they should be made with pasteurised egg, which removes any risk of salmonella. Cheesecakes are sometimes made with ricotta or mascarpone cheese, both of which are safe to eat during pregnancy.

✗ You should avoid eating homemade cheesecakes that are not cooked. These contain gelatine and are put in the fridge to set. They carry the risk of salmonella as they contain uncooked eggs. If you are unsure about how a homemade cheesecake or one in a restaurant has been made, it is best to ask.

✓ **Cheese spread** Processed cheese spread, such as Dairylea, Laughing Cow, Primula and similar own-brand products from supermarkets, are fine to eat. Also see *cream cheese*.

✓ **Chicken** Provides a good source of protein, iron and B vitamins. It is important to check that it is cooked thoroughly until the juices run clear before eating, otherwise it can cause salmonella food poisoning. See page 25 for more on salmonella.

Chillies See *spicy food*.

✓ **Chocolate** A study in Finland found that mothers who ate chocolate regularly when they were pregnant had babies who smiled and laughed more.

Avoid eating too much chocolate, however, as it contains caffeine ✖
(50 mg per 50-g bar) as well as sugar and fat, which can contribute
to a high weight gain.

Chocolate mousse See *Mousse*.

Cider vinegar/apple cider vinegar To treat morning sickness, some ✔
people recommend putting a few drops or a teaspoonful of cider
vinegar into a glass of cold or warm water. This remedy seems to be
more popular in the USA than the UK. Advocates believe that sip-
ping this with meals or throughout the day will help reduce nausea.
A teaspoon of honey can be added to make it taste better. It is also
thought to be effective for heartburn or acid reflux. There is no scientific evidence that it is effective, but some women believe it
helps and there is certainly no harm in trying.

Some enthusiasts believe only unpasteurised apple cider vinegar ✖
is effective. However, this is best avoided because of the risk of
food poisoning.

Coffee It is safe to drink coffee during pregnancy and while breast- ✔ ✖
feeding, but you shouldn't have more than about two to three mugs
of instant coffee or two cups of real coffee a day. Other kinds of
coffee can contain much higher levels of caffeine. Also see the information on caffeine on page 30.

Cola It is safe to drink cola before or during pregnancy, and while ✔ ✖
breastfeeding, but you shouldn't have too much. It contains about
40 mg of caffeine per 330-ml can, so you need to count it alongside
tea and coffee (see page 30). Regular (not diet) varieties also contain
about 140 kcal per can, so if you drink large quantities you may gain excess weight without giving your baby the vitamins and minerals he or
she needs. Diet, light and lite varieties contain the same amount of
caffeine as regular colas, unless you specifically choose a caffeine-
free product. Diet colas also contain artificial sweeteners instead of
sugar, and some research suggests that intake of these should be kept
to a minimum during pregnancy and while breastfeeding.

✓ **Coleslaw** It is fine to eat coleslaw that is freshly made with salad cream or mayonnaise from a jar. Once coleslaw has been prepared, it should be stored in the fridge. Readymade coleslaw sold in the UK is also considered safe by the FSA. In some other counties, including the USA and Australia, women are advised to avoid pre-prepared coleslaw, particularly when sold at deli counters, because of the risk of listeria.

✗ Coleslaw prepared using homemade mayonnaise should be avoided as it contains raw eggs and therefore could result in salmonella poisoning.

✓ **Columbus eggs** These are safe to eat during pregnancy providing you follow the general advice about cooking until both the white and the yolk are solid (see *eggs*). Two eggs provide more than 220 mg of beneficial long-chain omega 3 fatty acids, so including them in your diet while you are pregnant or breastfeeding will boost your baby's supply.

✓ **Cottage cheese** It is fine to eat cottage cheese during pregnancy. However, avoid buying it from a delicatessen counter.

✓ **Crab** It is OK to eat crab if it is cooked properly and eaten hot, for example, crab cakes or crab and sweetcorn soup. It is also fine to eat cold crab if you are sure that it has been freshly cooked and cooled.

✗ It is best to avoid crab that is served cold if you are unsure about how recently is has been cooked and how it has been stored. Otherwise it could be contaminated with listeria or other food poisoning bacteria.

Crab sticks See *seafood sticks*.

Crayfish See *shellfish*.

Cream It is safe to eat all types of cream, including soured cream, ✓
clotted cream and crème fraiche, provided it is made from pasteurised milk. Raw or unpasteurised cream is not widely available
but is sold at some farmers' markets and specialist farm shops.
Cream, and products such as cream cakes that contain raw cream,
are legally required to give a warning on the packaging.

Cream cheese Products such as Philadelphia and similar own- ✓
brand soft cheese are safe to eat during pregnancy.

Crème anglaise See *custard*.

Crème brûlée It is generally safe to eat crème brûlée sold in super- ✓
markets and other shops as it is made from pasteurised eggs.

Homemade crème brûlée contains partially cooked eggs and should ✖
be avoided. In a restaurant, it is best to ask how it has been made.

Crème caramel It is safe to eat the kind of crème caramel that is ✓
sold in individual tubs in supermarkets, as it is made from pasteurised egg.

Homemade crème caramel contains partially cooked eggs and should ✖
be avoided. In a restaurant, it is best to ask how it has been made.

Crème fraiche See *cream*.

Cured meats For example, Parma ham, salami, prosciutto crudo, ✖
chorizo, Serrano ham and pepperoni. These are not cooked but are
preserved by salting and smoking, or by treating with sodium nitrite and nitrate. There is a small risk of catching toxoplasmosis
(see page 24), as there is with any uncooked meat.

Some 'cured ham' or 'dry-cured ham' is roasted or baked after cur- ✓
ing, in which case it is safe to eat. However, if there is no mention of
cooking on the label, then you should assume that it is not cooked.

Curry See *spicy food*.

✔ **Custard** It is fine to eat custard from a tin, long-life UHT ready-made custard sold in a carton, chilled custard sold in a supermarket described as 'fresh custard', and custard prepared by mixing custard powder with milk (providing it's pasteurised milk). All these products are made with pasteurised egg. It is also fine to eat egg custard tarts and custard slices sold in supermarkets.

✘ Homemade custard prepared using fresh eggs should not be eaten, as the eggs are only partially cooked and therefore could contain salmonella. In restaurants this is sometimes called crème anglaise – if you see it on a menu, it is best to ask whether it has been made with pasteurised eggs, and if not, it is best avoided.

✘ **Deli foods** The advice in the USA, Australia and New Zealand is not to eat food from delicatessen shops or counters if you are pregnant. The UK has no specific guidelines. However, it would be sensible to choose pre-packaged food rather than deli products whenever possible. This is because unpackaged foods can become contaminated with listeria from other products. Low-risk foods such as ham may have been handled with the same utensils used on higher-risk foods such as salami. In addition, you have no way of knowing whether deli foods are beyond their use-by date.

✔✘ **Diet drinks** The occasional can of diet cola or other drink is very unlikely to do any harm during pregnancy or while breastfeeding. However, no one knows whether a high intake of artificial sweeteners could have long-term effects, and so moderation is sensible. See also *artificial sweeteners*.

✔ **Dips** Pre-packaged dips such as houmous, tzatziki, salsa and sour cream or yogurt-based products should be safe to eat during pregnancy.

Dips sold at a deli counter are best avoided because of the risk of ✖
cross-contamination and less certainty about the use-by date. Any
dips containing blue cheese should be avoided.

Edam It is fine to eat Edam cheese during pregnancy. ✔

Egg nog As well as alcohol, fresh egg nog contains uncooked egg, ✖
which could contain salmonella. Best avoided.

Eggs Pregnant women should avoid eggs that are raw or partially ✖
cooked, as they may contain salmonella bacteria. Foods likely to
contain raw or only partially cooked eggs include:

- homemade mayonnaise;
- Béarnaise sauce and Hollandaise sauce;
- Caesar salad dressing and similar salad dressings;
- homemade puddings such as ice cream, mousse, cheesecake, tiramisu and lemon meringue pie;
- homemade royal icing, e.g. on a Christmas or wedding cake;
- homemade custard.

Organic eggs are just as likely to contain salmonella as free-range,
barn fresh or any other type of egg.

It is safe to eat eggs that are cooked until both the white and the ✔
yolk are solid. This will destroy any salmonella that might be present. So, you can have boiled, fried or scrambled eggs if they are
cooked thoroughly.

It is important to keep raw eggs away from other foods and to wash
your hands and any utensils after handling raw eggs to avoid cross-
contamination. Pasteurisation kills salmonella, and so it is generally
safe to eat commercially produced foods containing egg, as it is almost always pasteurised. This includes foods such as mayonnaise,
ice cream and mousse.

In restaurants, watch out for sauces and desserts that may contain eggs that are not completely cooked. If you are eating out and are unsure, it is best to ask.

British Lion Quality eggs (those stamped with a red lion) come from British hens that have been vaccinated against salmonella. If you buy these from a reputable shop, store them in the fridge and eat them well before the use-by date, then the risk of salmonella is extremely small. However, they are not guaranteed to be salmonella-free. If you eat dishes containing uncooked eggs away from home, then the risk is much higher. In a 2007 survey of caterers, it was found that half didn't refrigerate their eggs and 20% of samples were older than recommended.

Also see *Columbus eggs*.

✖ **Eggs Benedict** This dish contains poached eggs, which have a runny yolk, and hollandaise sauce, which is made with only partially cooked eggs. It should be avoided, as it could contain salmonella.

✔✖ **Energy drinks** If you are feeling tired and in need of a pick-me-up, an energy drink may seem like the answer. However, most have added caffeine or guarana (which also contains caffeine). Just like coffee or cola, these drinks count towards your daily caffeine limit of 300 mg per day during pregnancy (see page 30). Some energy drinks also contain herbs that could affect you or your baby. It is best to avoid them if you are unsure.

✔ **Fennel tea** Some breastfeeding mothers drink tea made from fennel, sometimes combined with other ingredients, to improve their milk supply. There is no scientific evidence that it works, but some women believe that it helps. It will not do any harm, so if you think your milk supply is low it may be worth trying fennel tea, as well as making sure that you are drinking plenty of fluids, resting and following the general advice for breastfeeding (see page 117). See *herbal teas* for information about other teas to boost breast milk supply.

✔ **Feta cheese** This is safe to eat during pregnancy.

Fish Women who are pregnant, breastfeeding or planning a pregnancy are advised to eat at least two portions of fish a week, including one portion of oily fish. A portion is about 140 g of cooked fish, which is equivalent to about 170 g before cooking. When you eat fish, make sure that it is cooked properly to avoid the risk of food poisoning.

It is safe to eat white fish during pregnancy, e.g. cod, coley, haddock, halibut, monkfish, mullet (red or grey), plaice, pollack, red snapper, sea bass, skate, sole, tilapia and turbot. White fish is low in fat and provides lots of protein, iodine, niacin and selenium. There is no limit set on the amount you can eat.

Oily fish such as anchovies, hake, herring, kipper, mackerel, pilchards, sprats, salmon, sardines, trout and whitebait are great for your baby's brain and eye development. However, oily fish may contain traces of pollutants, so you shouldn't eat more than two portions a week. See *oily fish* and omega 3s (page 97).

You should avoid eating shark, swordfish or marlin if you are pregnant or planning a pregnancy. They have been found to contain traces of mercury, which could affect your unborn baby's developing nervous system. If you are breastfeeding, you shouldn't eat more than one portion of these a week.

Tuna has also been found to contain mercury, but in much lower amounts. You shouldn't eat more than two portions of fresh tuna or four cans of tuna a week if you are pregnant or planning a pregnancy. There is no limit on the amount of tuna you can eat while breastfeeding. See *tuna*.

Also see *sushi* and *smoked fish*.

Fizzy drinks It is safe to drink the odd fizzy drink during pregnancy, but remember they generally contain sugar, which provides calories but none of the nutrients your baby needs. Some also contain artificial sweeteners, and both colas and energy drinks contain caffeine.

✓ **Flaxseeds** Also known as linseeds, these are a good source of alpha-linolenic acid (ALA), which is one of the shorter-chain omega 3 fatty acids. To a limited extent, ALA can be converted to long-chain omega 3s (EPA and DHA), which are important for fetal brain and eye development (see page 36).

Flaxseeds have a tough seed coating, so for maximum benefit they should be ground or at least crushed, otherwise the ALA-rich oil inside them is unavailable for absorption. Flaxseed oil is best eaten cold, for example in a salad dressing or added at the end of cooking, otherwise the ALA may become destabilised.

✓ **Fromage frais** It is safe to eat fromage frais during pregnancy.

✓ **Fruit** Fruit is an essential part of any healthy diet, but this is especially true if you are pregnant, breastfeeding or thinking about having a baby. Fruits are packed with vital vitamins, minerals and phytochemicals. You should aim to eat at least five portions of fruit and vegetables a day.

Some women find that acidic fruit, such as oranges, give them heartburn, especially during the later stages of pregnancy. If this is a problem for you, then avoid acidic fruit late in the day or completely for a while. If you are eating out and you have concerns about hygiene levels, it may be a good idea to avoid fruit salad and other pre-prepared fruit.

✓ **Fruit juice** Pure fruit juice counts as one of your five recommended portions of fruit and vegetables a day – but no matter how much you drink, it can never count as more than one portion. This is because it doesn't contain as much fibre as whole fruits do, and when the juice is being extracted some of the sugar is broken down into a form that can damage your teeth. Fruit juice makes a good alternative to tea, coffee and alcoholic drinks during pregnancy, but it does contain sugar, and therefore calories, so avoid drinking large amounts. It is always healthier to buy 100% pure fruit juice rather than a 'juice drink', which may contain only a small amount of fruit juice as well as sugar, artificial sweeteners and other additives.

Some women find that if they drink large quantities of orange juice while breastfeeding, their baby develops diarrhoea. If this happens, you should cut down on the amount of juice you drink. However, there is no need to avoid orange juice while breastfeeding just in case.

During pregnancy, you should drink only pasteurised fruit juice or juice ✗ you have squeezed at home yourself. Unpasteurised juice can be a source of listeria or *E. coli*. Most juices bought in supermarkets are pasteurised, even those that are sold chilled and described as 'freshly squeezed'. However, freshly squeezed juice bought from street stalls, farmers' markets and farm shops may not be pasteurised.

Garlic Eating garlic while breastfeeding has been shown to affect ✓ the flavour of breast milk. This isn't a problem and there is no need to avoid garlic unless your baby seems to dislike the flavour or has an adverse reaction such as an upset stomach (see page 123).

Ginger Ginger is a traditional remedy for morning sickness and ✓ nausea during pregnancy. Several trials have been conducted in Australia and Thailand in recent years to test its effectiveness. These have found that taking about 1g of ginger a day (or an equivalent amount in a capsule or syrup) is effective at reducing feelings of nausea and episodes of vomiting in the majority of women.

There are several ways to eat ginger: grated in stir-fries, soups and sauces, in biscuits and cakes, crystallised ginger, ginger marmalade, ginger beer and ginger ale (non-alcoholic). You can also make ginger tea by grating a little into a cup and adding boiling water. Some people find that adding lemon and honey makes this more palatable.

Goats' cheese There are several different types of goats' cheese ✗ available. When we think of goats' cheese, we usually mean Chèvre. This is a soft cheese with a white rind, similar to Brie. Like other mould-ripened cheeses, it should be avoided in pregnancy because of the risk of listeria. However, if it is cooked thoroughly and eaten hot, any listeria will be destroyed.

✓ It is fine to eat hard Cheddar-type cheeses made from goats' milk. It is also fine to eat soft goats' cheese if it is made from pasteurised milk and doesn't have a rind, as this means it is not mould-ripened.

✗ **Gravlax** Also called gravadlax (Swedish) and gravlaks (Norwegian). This is raw salmon that has been pickled or marinated, usually with salt and dill. It looks similar to smoked salmon, but it is not actually smoked. In Scandinavian countries, where it is more commonly consumed, pregnant women are advised that smoked salmon is safe to eat but cured fish, such as gravlax, shouldn't be eaten. There is no official advice regarding the safety of eating gravlax during pregnancy in the UK.

✓✗ **Green tea** Green tea is rich in antioxidants and may protect against heart disease and certain cancers. However, there is some suggestion that drinking large amounts around the time of conception may increase the risk of neural tube defects. This is because the anti-cancer compound epigallocatechin gallate (EGCG) found in green tea lowers folic acid levels. The evidence for this is not strong, but if you are pregnant or trying for a baby it would be sensible to limit your intake to no more than about two cups a day.

✓ **Gruyére cheese** It is fine to eat Gruyére cheese during pregnancy.

✗ **Guarana** This is a seed extract originally found in the Amazon. It contains caffeine and related compounds and is added to some energy drinks, herbal drinks and chewing gum. It is not advisable to take it during pregnancy or while breastfeeding as it is a stimulant and the effects on your baby are unknown.

✗ **Guinness** Along with other kinds of stout, Guinness was once thought to be good for pregnancy because it had lots of iron and would 'build you up'. However, Guinness contains only about 0.01mg of iron per 100ml, or 0.3mg per half-pint, compared with 3–7mg in a typical bowl of breakfast cereal. It also contains alcohol of course and so is not good for pregnancy or breastfeeding.

Halloumi cheese It is fine to eat halloumi cheese during pregnancy. ✔

Ham It is fine to eat pre-packaged cooked ham during pregnancy. ✔ This is often described as baked, boiled or honey-roasted ham.

Parma ham and other cured meats should be avoided because of ✖ the risk of toxoplasmosis. It may also be wise to avoid ham bought from deli counters, as there is an increased risk of listeria from cross-contamination from other, higher-risk foods.

Herbal teas These include any tea made from roots, berries, flowers, seeds or leaves other than tea leaves. Women may choose to take them during pregnancy and while breastfeeding to reduce their caffeine intake. Some herbal teas are recommended for pregnancy-related symptoms such as nausea, including peppermint and ginger teas. Others are thought to increase milk supply, for example fenugreek, aniseed, raspberry leaf and nettle. If you buy a herbal tea, make sure it is from a reputable source. It should contain a full list of all ingredients and be labelled with the manufacturer's and distributor's details and a best-before date.

It is fine to drink peppermint tea and ginger tea during pregnancy and ✔ while breastfeeding. Fennel *tea* is also considered safe for breastfeeding. Fruit teas containing ingredients that you might normally eat (e.g. blackcurrant, lemon, orange) are also considered safe.

If you are pregnant, you shouldn't drink raspberry leaf tea before ✖ about 34 weeks of pregnancy.

If you are breastfeeding, you should avoid sage tea.

It is also sensible to avoid drinking any teas made from unfamiliar ingredients, such as black cohort, ginseng and pennyroyal. These should be treated as drugs or medicines rather than foods, as many contain active ingredients that pass through the placenta to your baby or into breast milk, in the same way that medicines do. It is best to seek professional advice regarding their safety.

✘ **Hollandaise sauce** This generally contains partially cooked egg yolk, so it should be avoided in pregnancy because of the risk of salmonella.

✔ **Honey** It is fine to eat honey during pregnancy and while breast-feeding. Honey very occasionally contains the bacterium *Clostridium botulinum*, which babies' intestines may be unable to cope with, resulting in infant botulism. For this reason, babies under 12 months shouldn't have honey. However, the intestines of adults, including pregnant women, are able to stop any botulinum bacteria from growing and causing any problems.

✔ **Houmous** It is fine to eat houmous during pregnancy.

✔ **Ice cream** It is fine to eat ice cream sold pre-packaged in tubs or individually from supermarkets or similar shops.

✘ Homemade ice cream generally contains raw or partially cooked eggs (just like custard). It should therefore be avoided in pregnancy, as it may contain salmonella.

Soft (Mr Whippy type) ice cream from kiosks and ice cream vans should be avoided because of the risk of listeria if machinery isn't kept scrupulously clean.

✔ **Jarlsberg** It is safe to eat Jarlsberg cheese during pregnancy.

Juice See *fruit juice*.

Lemon curd Commercially prepared lemon curd bought from a supermarket is fine to eat during pregnancy. ✔

Homemade lemon curd contains partially cooked eggs and should ✘
be avoided in pregnancy because of the risk of salmonella.

Lemon juice Some women report that a tablespoon of lemon juice ✔
is an effective natural remedy for heartburn. There is no scientific
evidence to support this, but it's perfectly safe and worth a try.

Lettuce It is safe to eat lettuce during pregnancy, provided that you ✔ ✘
wash it thoroughly. You should even wash pre-washed salad leaves
bought in bags, in order to avoid the risk of listeria and salmonella.

Liquorice It is fine to eat liquorice in moderation during pregnancy. ✔ ✘
However, consuming more than about 250 g a week is associated
with an increased risk of premature delivery (birth before 37
weeks). This was discovered in Finland, where liquorice is very popular
among young women. It is not understood why liquorice has
this effect, but it is probably related to its glycyrrhizin content.

Liver Liver and foods made from liver, such as liver pâté, should be ✘
avoided during pregnancy. They contain high levels of vitamin A in
the form of retinol, which can harm your baby's development (see
page 38). Previous generations of women were encouraged to eat
liver during pregnancy because of its high iron content, and this may
have been good advice at the time. However, animals now consume
feeds with a high vitamin A content, leading to increased levels of
the vitamin in their liver, so this advice is no longer appropriate.

It is fine to eat liver while you are breastfeeding. ✔

Mackerel This is an oily fish and a good source of long-chain omega ✔ ✘
3 fatty acids. However, you shouldn't have more than two portions
a week (140 g each). See also *fish* and *smoked mackerel*.

✓ **Mascarpone cheese** It is fine to eat mascarpone cheese during pregnancy.

✓ **Mayonnaise** It is safe to eat mayonnaise bought in a jar from a supermarket or similar shop during pregnancy. Mayonnaises sold at room temperature (rather than chilled) are made with pasteurised egg.

✗ During pregnancy, you should avoid homemade mayonnaise as it contains raw unpasteurised egg and could potentially contain salmonella. Occasionally, fresh mayonnaise containing unpasteurised eggs is sold in shops and at markets. You can usually recognise this, because it's sold chilled and has a relatively soon use-by date.

✓ **Meat** Most meat and poultry is fine, as long as it's cooked properly. Similarly, if you're eating a ready meal, it's important to make sure it is heated properly so that it is piping hot all the way through.

✗ Don't eat raw or undercooked meat, as it may contain salmonella, campylobacter, toxoplasmosis or *E.coli*. This means rare steak, Parma ham, salami and similar products are out.

To avoid cross-contamination from raw to cooked meat, store them separately and covered, use different knives, chopping boards and other utensils, and wash your hands carefully after handling raw meat.

✓ **Meringue** Meringues sold in supermarkets and similar shops should be safe to eat during pregnancy, as they are generally prepared using pasteurised eggs. It is also safe to eat homemade meringues that are hard, for example a Pavlova or meringue nest, if it has been cooked properly and is no longer sticky in the middle. The core temperature should reach 70 °C for two minutes to ensure that any salmonella that might be present are killed. If normal cooking instructions are followed and the meringue is cooked for two to three hours at about 110 °C, this shouldn't be a problem.

✗ Soft meringue that has only been browned in the oven should be avoided, as the egg white isn't cooked properly and there is a potential risk of salmonella. This means that puddings such as home-made lemon meringue pie and baked Alaska should be avoided.

Milk During pregnancy, it is safe to drink milk provided it has been ✔
heat-treated to kill any harmful bacteria. This means that you can have pasteurised, UHT, sterilised and dried milk. It is safe to drink whole milk, semi-skimmed and skimmed milk provided it has been heat-treated in one of these ways. Likewise, you could drink goats' or ewes' milk instead of cows' milk if it has been heat-treated. It is also safe to drink evaporated milk and condensed milk.

For pregnant and breastfeeding women, milk and milk products such as cheese and yogurt are an important part of the diet. They provide protein, calcium and vitamins B_{12} and D. Milk can also help relieve the symptoms of heartburn. It is recommended that you have one or two portions a day, but whenever possible choose lower-fat options, such as semi-skimmed milk and low-fat yogurt. Consuming less than one cup of milk a day is associated with a small reduction in birth weight. If you don't drink milk or eat milk products, you need to get the nutrients they provide from other sources (see Chapter 3).

It is best to avoid drinking unpasteurised milk (including goats' milk ✘
and sheep's milk) and using it in cooking while you are pregnant. Un-pasteurised milk may contain listeria and other bacteria, such as *E. coli* and brucella, which can cause food poisoning.

Also see *organic milk*.

Monkey nuts See *peanuts*.

Mousse It is safe to eat mousse bought from a supermarket or ✔
large retailer while you are pregnant. If it contains any egg, it should be pasteurised.

Homemade mousse usually contains raw egg and should be ✘
avoided in pregnancy because of the risk of salmonella.

✔ **Mozzarella** It is safe to eat mozzarella cheese during pregnancy, whether it is made from pasteurised or unpasteurised milk.

✘ **Mud** If you have a craving for mud or earth, this is one that you shouldn't satisfy. By eating bits of mud, even if it's just very muddy potatoes, you risk toxoplasmosis, listeria and other forms of food poisoning. See the section on cravings on page 10.

✔ **Mussels** It is OK to eat mussels if they are cooked properly and served as part of a piping hot dish, such as moules marinière, seafood soup or fish pie. Canned mussels are also OK.

✘ It is best to avoid mussels served cold, unless you are sure they have been freshly cooked and chilled.

✔✘ **Nitrites** Nitrates and nitrites are added to cured meats and fish as a preservative (to prevent bacterial growth) and to produce their characteristic pink or red colour. They are generally added to ham, salami, bacon, corned beef, hotdogs and smoked mackerel. To identify foods containing nitrites, look on the food label for potassium nitrate, potassium nitrite, sodium nitrate, sodium nitrite and saltpetre, or the E numbers for these additives (E249 to E252).

Concern has been raised about these preservatives because they are converted to nitroso compounds in the body. These have been shown to cause cancer when given in large doses to animals, and it is suspected that they could have the same effect in humans. One study found that women with a high intake of cured meat (more than 100 g per day throughout pregnancy) were more likely to have children who developed childhood brain tumours. Other, similar studies have not found the same effect, but it seems sensible to consume cured meats and similar products containing nitrites only in moderation during pregnancy. It is not known whether nitrites pass into breast milk, so moderation is advisable while breastfeeding as well.

Nutmeg It is fine to eat nutmeg in normal cooking, for example in ✔ cakes, biscuits and rice pudding.

Large quantities of ground nutmeg and nutmeg oil, which is some- ✖ times used in aromatherapy, should be avoided during pregnancy. These can result in hallucinations and palpitations in the mother and increased fetal heart rate.

Nuts It is OK to eat almonds, Brazil nuts, hazelnuts, pecans, wal- ✔ nuts and other kinds of nut while you are pregnant, unless you are allergic to them. This applies whether you are pregnant, trying for a baby or breastfeeding.

If you have a family history of allergic conditions, the current ad- ✖ vice is to avoid peanuts during pregnancy and while breastfeeding (Also see *peanuts*).

Oily fish Women who are pregnant, breastfeeding or trying for a ✔ ✖ baby should have one or two portions of oily fish a week, according to the FSA. Oily fish such as salmon and sardines is rich in beneficial omega 3 fatty acids (see below) and provides protein and essential vitamins and minerals. However, you shouldn't eat too much, as oily fish can contain high levels of dioxins and polychlorinated biphenols (PCBs). These are pollutants found widely in the environment but in higher concentrations in oily fish. Neither has an immediate effect on health, but high levels may cause problems in the long term.

You shouldn't let this put you off eating moderate amounts of oily fish. Dioxins and PCBs are impossible to avoid entirely as they are present in many other foods and are widespread in the environment. Exposure from dietary sources has fallen by about 75% in the past 20 years because of tighter controls on industrial pollution. Further- more, scientists have found that the benefits of eating oily fish far outweigh the possible risks associated with dietary exposure to dioxins and PCBs. After reviewing all the evidence, two expert com- mittees (the Scientific Advisory Committee on Nutrition and the Committee on Toxicology) concluded in 2004 that, during pregnancy and while breastfeeding, the benefits outweigh the risks if women consume one or two portions a week. Some experts believe that the limits should be raised. A study of more than 5000 women in the Bristol area found that children's development (including scores for social development and dexterity in skills such as drawing at age three years and verbal IQ scores at age eight years) benefited most when their mothers consumed more than 340g of seafood per week during pregnancy (which is nearly two and a half portions a week).

See *fish, tuna* and page 37 for more on the benefits of omega 3s.

✔ **Omelette** It is fine to eat omelettes during pregnancy providing you ensure that the egg is cooked until completely set. Check in particular that it is not runny in the centre.

✔✖ **Oregano** It is safe to use oregano in cooking while you are pregnant. However, when oregano is added to a meal, it reduces the amount of iron your body absorbs, so it is best not to use it regularly, particularly if you have low or borderline iron levels.

✖ Oregano oil (used in aromatherapy) is considered a uterine stimulant and should be avoided in pregnancy.

✔ **Organic food** Eating organic food reduces your consumption of fertiliser and pesticide residues. Organic food is also free from genetically modified (GM) ingredients and contains a much smaller range of food additives. It may also contain higher levels of certain nutrients and flavonoids, but this hasn't been established firmly.

Nobody knows whether eating organic food during pregnancy or while breastfeeding is really better for your baby. Some people claim that going organic could reduce the risks of childhood cancer and early puberty, or benefit cognitive development, but there just isn't the scientific evidence to back this up. All chemicals used in food, including pesticides sprayed on crops and colourings added to processed foods, are tested for safety, and there is nothing to suggest that these are harmful to babies' development. However, hundreds of new chemicals have been introduced to the food system in the past 60 to 100 years and no one knows what long-term effects may be uncovered in the years to come. Many women choose to eat organic food as a precaution to reduce the amount of chemicals they, and therefore their baby, are exposed to.

If you eat organic food, you need to be just as careful about washing all fruit and vegetables before eating, in order to avoid exposure to harmful bacteria. You should also remember that just because something is organic, it isn't necessarily healthy. Organic cola is still sugary water containing caffeine and a few other additives, and organic carrot cake and chocolate still, unfortunately, contain lots of calories. Also, organic food products are not fortified with extra vitamins and minerals. Therefore, if you eat foods such as organic breakfast cereals, you may have a lower intake of certain nutrients, such as iron and B vitamins.

Organic milk Pasteurised organic milk is safe to drink when you ✔ are pregnant or breastfeeding (see *milk* for further information). The levels of omega 3 fatty acids in organic milk are higher than those in conventional milk. However, milk contains ALA, which is a short-chain omega 3 fatty acid. It is the long-chain omega 3s (found in oily fish) that are particularly important for fetal brain and eye development. Although the body can convert short-chain omega 3s to long-chain omega 3s, the conversion appears limited. This means that organic milk shouldn't be considered a substitute for oily fish.

Oysters Oysters are usually eaten raw and should be avoided be- ✘ cause of the risk of food poisoning. Like other raw shellfish, they can, very occasionally, contain hepatitis A (see *shellfish*). They can also contain a virus called the norovirus, which can result in nausea, diarrhoea, abdominal pain, headache and fever.

✔ **Papaya** (pawpaw) Papaya is a good source of vitamin A (as beta-carotene) and vitamin C and there is no need to avoid it while you are pregnant or breastfeeding. In the past, particularly in parts of Asia, it was believed that eating papaya during pregnancy could cause miscarriage. Papaya contains an enzyme called papain, which breaks down proteins and helps to tenderise meat. This may have something to do with the traditional beliefs, but there is no evidence that normal consumption presents any cause for concern.

✘ **Parma ham** (prosciutto do Parma, prosciutto crudo) This is not cooked and should be avoided during pregnancy (see *cured meat*).

✔ **Parmesan cheese** This is considered safe to eat during pregnancy, whether it is made from pasteurised or unpasteurised milk. This is because it is acidic and has a low moisture content, so it isn't a suitable environment for bacteria such as listeria to grow.

✔ **Parsley** This is safe to eat in normal cooking.

✘ Consuming extremely large quantities of parsley should be avoided as this could have a uterine stimulant effect.

✘ **Pâté** Any pâté containing liver should be avoided during pregnancy, as it contains high levels of vitamin A (see *liver*). Other types of fresh pâté, including vegetable pâté, should also be avoided as they may contain listeria.

✔ It is safe to eat pâté (except liver pâté) that is tinned or pasteurised while you are pregnant.

Pâté (all types) is considered safe while breastfeeding.

✔ **Pavlova** It is OK to eat Pavlova during pregnancy, provided the meringue is cooked until solid right through to the centre. See also *meringue*.

Peanuts Also known as groundnuts and monkey nuts. The current ✖
government advice is to avoid peanuts while pregnant or breastfeeding if you have a close family history of atopy. This means if
you, the baby's father or any of your or his children have allergies,
eczema, asthma or hay fever. It doesn't apply if it is only other relatives, such as your parents or siblings, who are affected.

Avoidance during breastfeeding appears to be more important
than during pregnancy. However, the evidence regarding avoidance
is currently being reviewed, and the guidelines may well change in
the near future.

If you choose to avoid whole peanuts, you should also avoid products containing peanuts, such as peanut butter and cold-pressed
or unrefined/unprocessed (crude) peanut or groundnut oil. However, refined peanut oil is not thought to be a problem, as the
peanut proteins (which are responsible for allergies) are removed
during processing.

There is no evidence to suggest that other women should avoid ✔
peanuts while pregnant or breastfeeding. In fact, some evidence
suggests that avoidance in early life could actually increase the risk
of a person developing a peanut allergy.

Peppermint tea It is safe to drink peppermint tea during pregnancy. ✔
Some women find that it helps to relieve indigestion, heartburn,
nausea and morning sickness.

There is some suggestion, although no firm evidence, that drinking ✖
large quantities could cause miscarriage. As a precaution, it is probably best not to drink several very strong cups of peppermint tea
close together.

Pepperoni This is a type of dried sausage like salami or chorizo. It ✖
is uncooked and so should be avoided in pregnancy because of the
risk of toxoplasmosis.

✔ **Philadelphia cheese** During pregnancy, it is OK to eat Philadelphia cheese and other, similar brands of cream cheese.

✔ **Pineapple** You may have heard that pineapple should be avoided during pregnancy because it can cause miscarriage, or that you should eat it at the end of pregnancy to kick-start labour. The truth is that normal pineapple consumption is highly unlikely to have any effect at any stage of pregnancy.

Fresh pineapple contains an enzyme called bromelain, which breaks down proteins. In a highly concentrated tablet form, bromelain is used to treat inflammation. Taking bromelain tablets or capsules during pregnancy is not advised, as it may cause abnormal bleeding. However, some alternative therapists may recommend them for the end of pregnancy, to help the cervix soften and dilate more readily, although no evidence has been found that this is effective. To get enough bromelain from fresh pineapple to have any possible effect, you would need to eat between seven and ten fresh pineapples at one sitting. Tinned pineapple and pineapple juice contain little or no bromelain.

✔ **Pine nuts** (pine kernels) Pine nuts are safe to eat unless you have a specific allergy to them. There is no evidence that avoidance during pregnancy or while breastfeeding will reduce the risk of your child developing a nut allergy or any other form of allergy.

✔ **Pizza** It is generally safe to eat any kind of pizza where all of the topping is cooked properly. This includes pizzas made with goats' cheese, Stilton, Gorgonzola and any other kind of cheese, provided that it is cooked until piping hot. These cheeses could contain listeria, but it would be killed by proper cooking.

✘ Pizzas topped with Parma ham should be avoided as the ham is added after cooking and there is a risk of food poisoning (see *cured meat*).

Port Salut cheese It is fine to eat Port Salut while you are pregnant. ✔

Potato salad It is safe to eat homemade potato salad during preg- ✔
nancy provided it is made with mayonnaise from a jar. It is also safe
to eat commercially prepared potato salad sold in supermarkets
and similar shops.

Potato salad made with homemade mayonnaise should be avoided ✖
during pregnancy, as it contains raw eggs and could be contaminated with salmonella. Potato salad from delicatessens and any
that is left out for several hours at a barbeque or on a buffet table
is best avoided because of the risk of listeria.

Prawns It is safe to eat prawns that are cooked properly and ✔
served as part of a hot meal, for example in a curry or stir-fry. Cold
prawns in a salad or sandwich should be safe if they have been
cooked and then chilled and kept cold until they are eaten.

If you have any doubts about how cold prawns have been cooked ✖
or stored, they are best avoided because of the risk of food poisoning (see *shellfish*).

Prebiotics These are food ingredients that aren't digested directly ✔
but are consumed by so-called 'friendly bacteria' in the large intestine. They help the beneficial bacteria in the gut to multiply at the
expense of potentially harmful bacteria. There is nothing to suggest that prebiotics, such as galacto-oligosaccharides, shouldn't
be consumed while you are pregnant or breastfeeding. There is
little research so far, but they may be beneficial.

Probiotics These are live micro-organisms that are beneficial to ✔
health. It is safe to drink products containing probiotics during
pregnancy and while breastfeeding. If a food or drink containing
probiotics is not safe for pregnancy, then it will carry a warning saying so. If you are thinking of taking a probiotic supplement, rather
than a food or drink containing probiotics, check carefully what

other ingredients it contains. Some probiotic supplements contain vitamins and minerals, as well as probiotics, and these may be at levels that are not suitable for pregnancy.

There is some evidence that exposure to particular probiotics around the time of birth is protective against allergies (see page 4). In addition, it appears that taking probiotics during pregnancy may help with constipation and in the treatment of vaginal infections, which are sometimes associated with premature labour.

✖ **Prosciutto** This is the Italian word for ham, but in English it usually means smoked spiced Italian ham. Prosciutto is cured but not cooked, and it should be avoided during pregnancy because of the risk of toxoplasmosis.

✔ **Prunes** Prunes and prune juice are age-old remedies for constipation. Their laxative effect cannot be explained completely by fibre – prunes contain similar amounts of fibre as other dried fruits, and prune juice contains no fibre at all, as it is filtered before bottling. The unique effect is more likely to be due to the high levels of sorbitol that prunes contain, which is a type of sugar that is absorbed very slowly and can pass into the large intestine like fibre. Prunes also contain large amounts of phenolic compounds, which can also have a natural laxative effect.

Pu-Erh tea This is the tea reported to have helped Victoria Beckham regain her pre-pregnancy figure. Among the health benefits attributed to it are an ability to melt fat and reduce blood cholesterol levels. There is no evidence to back up these claims or other beliefs that it raises metabolism and aids weight loss. The best way to lose weight after having a baby is sensible eating and regular exercise (see page 122). Also, drinking tea with meals is not recommended, as it reduces your absorption of much needed micro-nutrients, particularly iron.

Quiche Commercially prepared quiche should be safe to eat dur- ✓
ing pregnancy. If you are in any doubt, rather than eating it cold,
heat it according to the manufacturer's guidelines and ensure that
it is hot all the way through. Homemade quiche should also be
cooked carefully to ensure the egg becomes solid.

Quorn™ All Quorn products contain mycoprotein, which is suitable ✓
for vegetarians. Unlike tofu, which is derived from soya, mycoprotein is part of the fungi family, like mushrooms. Quorn products are
a good source of vegetable protein, are low in fat and also provide
fibre. There is nothing to suggest that Quorn products are not suitable during pregnancy or while breastfeeding.

Raspberry leaf tea Taking raspberry leaf tea in the later stages of ✓
pregnancy is thought to help prepare the womb for labour. Raspberry
leaf is available as a tea and in tablet form from most health food
shops. Raspberry leaf is a uterine stimulant and is thought to
strengthen the muscles of the womb, so that when you have contrac-
tions they are more effective and labour is easier. In an Australian
study, women were given two raspberry leaf supplements per day
(1.2 g each) from 32 weeks of pregnancy. The second stage of labour
(pushing the baby out) was ten minutes shorter on average for these
women than for those receiving a placebo. They also had a lower rate
of forceps delivery (19% versus 30%). There is no evidence that
raspberry leaf tea will bring on labour, even if your baby is overdue.

It is not advisable to take raspberry leaf tea before 32 weeks of ✗
pregnancy, as you don't want to stimulate the uterine muscles before the baby is ready to be born.

Red Bull See *energy drinks*.

Red wine sauce It is fine to have red wine gravy and foods such as ✓
pears poached in red wine while pregnant or breastfeeding. A single serving will contain so little alcohol that it's not worth worrying

about. Most recipes use very little wine anyway, and much of the alcohol is cooked off. It is estimated that after 15 minutes of cooking, 60% of the alcohol is lost; after an hour, 75% is lost.

✓ **Rice** It is generally safe to eat rice, but take care with rice salads and dishes containing re-heated rice, such as kedgeree, biriyani and egg-fried rice. Rice can contain spores of *Bacillus cereus* bacteria, which can germinate if the dish is left standing at room temperature. The longer rice is left, the more these bacteria will multiply. The bacteria produce toxins that can cause food poisoning (vomiting and diarrhoea). It is not known whether *Bacillus cereus* has any other effects during pregnancy.

It is best to eat rice that has just been cooked. Alternatively, it should be cooled down within an hour, stored in the fridge and eaten within 24 hours. When re-heating rice, make sure it is piping hot all the way through.

✓ **Ricotta** It is fine to eat ricotta cheese in pregnancy.

✗ **Roquefort cheese** This is a blue cheese and should be avoided during pregnancy because of the risk of listeria.

✓ It is fine to eat a dish such as steak with Roquefort sauce, if it is cooked until bubbling hot, as this will kill any listeria present.

Saccharin See *artificial sweeteners*.

✓ **Sage** It is fine to eat foods containing sage while you are pregnant or breastfeeding.

✗ Sage is thought to have an oestrogen-like effect and may stimulate the uterus when taken in large quantities, so sage oil (used in aromatherapy) should be avoided during pregnancy. If you are breastfeeding, sage tea should be avoided, as it may interfere with milk production. However, if you want to stop breastfeeding, drinking sage tea may help to reduce the amount of milk you are producing and therefore ease any discomfort.

Salad Salads are a healthy option, but it is important that all ingre- ✔
dients are washed well to reduce the risk of food poisoning. Pre-
packaged salad bought in bags should be washed, even if it is labelled
as washed and ready to eat. This is because such bags have very occasionally been found to be contaminated with listeria or salmonella.

If you are eating out, particularly if you are travelling abroad, it is ✖
best to avoid salads unless you are completely confident about the
levels of hygiene.

See also *coleslaw* and *potato salad*.

Salami This should be avoided during pregnancy because it isn't ✖
cooked and could be contaminated with toxoplasmosis. See also
cured meat.

Salmon Salmon is safe and healthy in reasonable quantities. It pro- ✔ ✖
vides protein, iron and vitamins B_6, B_{12} and D. It also contains omega
3 fatty acids, which are beneficial for your baby. However, as all oily
fish contain traces of pollutants, you are advised not to eat more
than two portions a week. There has been some speculation about
whether farmed or wild salmon is better, but the FSA has concluded that there is no significant difference between the two. Wild
salmon has been found to contain higher levels of omega 3s, but
also higher levels of pollutants, than farmed salmon.

See also *smoked salmon, gravlax* and *oily fish*.

Sandwiches When you are making sandwiches at home, remember
to wash any salad ingredients. If you are buying a sandwich, go to a
shop or restaurant where you trust the level of hygiene. It may be
better to choose a pre-packaged sandwich rather than one prepared at a deli counter, where cross-contamination is more likely.

The following sandwiches should all be safe to eat: cheese and ✔
pickle, ploughman's, egg mayonnaise, ham salad, tuna and sweetcorn, chicken, houmous, poached salmon. If you have any doubts

about how sandwiches have been stored, for example whether they have been chilled from the time of preparation, it may be better to avoid sandwiches filled with prawn mayonnaise, crab or crayfish.

✘ Sandwiches filled with Brie or Stilton should be avoided.

✔ ✘ **Sardines** These are an oily fish and a good source of omega 3 fatty acids, iron, zinc and vitamin B$_{12}$. One small tin of sardines contains about two-thirds of a portion of oily fish. Therefore, you can eat up to three tins of sardines a week if you don't have any other oily fish.

✔ ✘ **Satay (saté)** Dishes such as satay pork, lamb or chicken are pre-pared with a peanut sauce. Therefore, they should be avoided if you have a family history of allergies (see *peanuts*). If not, they are fine to eat.

✔ **Scrambled eggs** It is fine to eat scrambled egg while you are preg-nant. However, make sure you cook the eggs well. If they are slightly runny, there is a risk of salmonella.

Seafood See *shellfish*.

✔ **Seafood sticks** These are sometimes referred to as crab sticks or fish sticks. They are usually made from processed white fish with crab flavouring, among other additives. They should be safe to eat, provided they are kept chilled.

✔ **Shellfish** It is OK to have shellfish such as prawns and mussels when you are pregnant, providing it is cooked thoroughly and eaten as part of a hot meal. For example, you could have shellfish in a fish pie, curry or stir-fry.

It is also safe to eat shellfish such as prawns or crab that has been freshly cooked and chilled. This means that products such as prawn sandwiches are OK if they are bought from a reputable shop and you are confident that the shellfish has been kept chilled from the time of cooking.

Shellfish such as oysters, whelks and cockles that is usually eaten raw should be avoided, as it can be contaminated with harmful bacteria and viruses, including hepatitis A.

It is also best to avoid shellfish that is cooked but served cold, for example prawn sandwiches and crab or lobster salad, if you have any doubts about the way it has been prepared or stored.

Raw or partially cooked shellfish can contain hepatitis A, which affects the liver. Symptoms include nausea, abdominal pain, tiredness, fever, dark urine and jaundice.

Smoked fish In the USA and Australia, pregnant women are advised not to eat smoked fish, including smoked salmon and mackerel, unless it is hot. This is because of the potential danger of listeria. However, the risk is low compared with foods such as Brie and pâté, and in the UK smoked fish is officially considered OK. That said, in 2007 there were two incidences where batches of smoked salmon were recalled by shops because of contamination with listeria.

Another issue that concerns some women is the polycyclic aromatic hydrocarbon (PAH) content of smoked fish. PAHs are present due to both sea pollution and the smoking process. Most PAHs are safe to consume, but some are believed to be carcinogenic. Levels of the carcinogenic PAHs benzo(a)pyrene have been found to be higher in fish smoked in traditional kilns than in fish smoked in larger commercial kilns. Smoked fish, like other smoked foods, also contains nitrates and nitrites, which are also potential carcinogens (see *nitrites*). Levels of salt are also usually high, and much higher than those in ordinary fish. These issues do not mean that smoked fish is completely out, because the real danger is not really known. However, it is best to consume smoked fish in moderation (see *oily fish* for portion limits), and satisfying a daily craving for smoked salmon bagels probably isn't a good idea.

✔ ✘ **Smoked mackerel** In the UK, it is considered safe to eat smoked mackerel during pregnancy (see *oily fish* for portion limits). See also *smoked fish*.

✔ ✘ **Smoked salmon** In the UK, it is considered safe to eat smoked salmon during pregnancy (see *oily fish* for portion limits). See *also gravlax* and *smoked fish*.

✔ **Soft cheese** See *cheese*.

✔ **Sour cream** It is OK to consume sour cream during pregnancy.

Soya There are no problems associated with eating soya beans or products such as tofu and soya milk, as part of a normal healthy diet. Concern has been raised about possible adverse effects that soya may have on fetal development, but these are not well founded. Soya contains a phytoestrogen called genistein, which can have a similar, but much weaker, effect as the hormone oestrogen. Research has shown that when pregnant rats consume a diet rich in genistein, it can affect the future fertility of their babies. It has been speculated that a diet rich in soya could have a similar effect in humans, but there is no evidence for this.

One study found that the incidence of hypospadius (a defect of the penis) was more common among babies of vegetarian mothers, and it was suggested that this could be related to a higher phytoestrogen intake. However, countries with a high intake of soya, such as China and Japan, do not appear to have such problems. Therefore, the balance of evidence suggests normal consumption is fine.

✔ **Spicy food** It's fine to eat spicy foods such as curry and chilli while you are pregnant, as long as you feel OK when you eat them. If you eat food that is too spicy, it can irritate the lining of the intestine and have a laxative effect. This is very unlikely to have a serious effect on your baby, but it will be unpleasant for you and will also leave you dehydrated.

It is sometimes suggested that eating a hot curry will bring on labour. However, this is probably one of those things that will help only if your baby is ready to come. If things have not started already, it's unlikely to have any effect (see page 16).

Spinach This is safe to eat and is a good source of beta-carotene, ✔ folate and vitamin C. However, it is a myth that spinach is a good source of iron: spinach contains oxalic acid, which binds tightly to the iron, making much of it unavailable for absorption.

Splenda® See *artificial sweeteners*.

Steak tartar (steak Americaine) This is a definite no-no during ✖ pregnancy. It contains raw meat, which could be infected with toxoplasmosis, and raw egg, so there is also a risk of salmonella.

Stilton This is a blue-veined cheese and should be avoided during ✖ pregnancy because of the risk of listeria.

It is OK to eat Stilton in a cooked dish that is piping hot, for exam- ✔ ple broccoli and Stilton soup, as this will kill any listeria that may be present.

Sucralose See *artificial sweeteners*.

Sulphites If you usually consume foods and drinks containing sul- ✔ phites, there is no reason to avoid them during pregnancy. Sulphites are additives (numbers E220 to E228) used to preserve food and prevent discolouration or browning in products such as dried apricots and sun-dried tomatoes. They are also found in sausages, burgers, soft drinks and wine. Some people are sensitive to sulphites and may have an asthmatic attack when exposed to them. Therefore, any food or drink containing sulphites carries a warning to alert these individuals.

✓ **Sushi** Raw fish is fine, as long as it's been frozen beforehand. Freezing kills off any tiny worms in the fish, which could otherwise make you ill. Readymade sushi brought into shops or restaurants should be safe, since food safety regulations state that it must have been frozen to –20°C for 24 hours. Restaurants that prepare their own fresh sushi may not have done this, so check with the staff. If you make sushi at home, freeze the fish for at least 24 hours before eating it.

✗ **Swordfish** High levels of mercury have been found in swordfish, and women who are pregnant are advised not to consume it at all. If you are breastfeeding, the advice is that it is OK to consume one portion a week but no more.

✓ **Taramasalata** Commercially prepared taramasalata is considered safe to eat during pregnancy by the FSA.

✓ **Tartar sauce** It is safe to eat tartar sauce from a jar or sachet, as this is made with pasteurised egg.

✗ Homemade tartar sauce is often prepared in the same way as homemade mayonnaise, in which case it will contain raw eggs and carry a risk of salmonella. However, it can also be made with hard-boiled egg yolks, which are safe, so it is best to ask.

✓ **Tea** It is fine to drink normal black tea in moderation. However, each cup contains about 50 mg of caffeine, so during pregnancy you shouldn't drink more than about six cups a day. If you like your tea strong, and drink large mugs, then the caffeine content will be higher. Also, if you drink coffee and cola as well, then you should have even fewer cups of tea (see page 30). You could try alternatives such as decaffeinated tea, peppermint tea or fruit teas.

✗ Try to avoid drinking tea (regular or decaffeinated) with meals or just after, as it can dramatically reduce iron absorption. The polyphenols in tea, known as tannins, bind tightly to the iron in foods such as breakfast cereal and bread, so the iron passes through your digestive system unabsorbed. Likewise, if you are taking iron supplements or multivitamins with iron, avoid drinking tea for about an hour after taking them.

See also *green tea, herbal teas, peppermint tea, pu-Erh tea* and *raspberry leaf tea*.

Thyme It is fine to use thyme in ordinary cooking. ✔

Strong medicinal doses of thyme and thyme essential oil should be ✖ avoided during pregnancy, as it is thought to be a uterine stimulant.

Tiramisu It is fine to eat tiramisu bought from a supermarket ✔ or similar shop while you are pregnant, as any egg it contains will be pasteurised.

Homemade tiramisu may contain raw eggs in the creamy topping, ✖ so it should be avoided because of the risk of salmonella. There are several recipes for making tiramisu without eggs, however, so if you are making your own, try one of these.

Tofu It is fine to eat tofu during pregnancy and while breastfeed- ✔ ing. See also *soya*.

Tuna It is safe to eat tuna in moderation. It is recommended that ✔ ✖ while pregnant you have no more than two portions of fresh tuna (140 g a portion) or four medium-sized cans per week. If you do have four cans of tuna in a week, you can still have two portions of oily fish, such as salmon or mackerel, but not fresh tuna.

Fresh tuna is an oily fish and provides omega 3 fatty acids, which are good for your baby's development. However, it can also contain pollutants (dioxins and PCBs). Tinned tuna is not considered an oily fish, since during the canning process much of the oil is separated and lost. As a result, tinned tuna has a similar fatty acid composition to white fish. This means that tinned tuna isn't a good source of omega

3 oils, and it is not a problem as far as PCBs are concerned. However, because both fresh and canned tuna have been found to contain mercury, they should be consumed only in moderation.

There is no limit on the amount of tuna you can eat while breast-feeding.

✔ **Water** All adults need to drink at least 1.2 litres of fluid a day, which is approximately six to eight glasses. While you are pregnant, you may notice that you become thirstier. Breastfeeding is definitely very thirsty work. If it's hot or you're exercising, you will need more fluids. Since it is not advisable to drink alcohol while pregnant, and your caffeine intake should be limited, water is an important part of your diet. Tap water is just as good as bottled water and its quality is closely monitored.

✖ **Wine** It is not advisable to drink wine during pregnancy. See the information on alcohol on page 26.

✔ **Yogurt** It is safe to eat yogurt while you are pregnant. This includes products described as 'bio-yogurts' or containing 'live bacteria'. The bacteria they contain are probiotics or 'healthy bacteria', so they will not cause food poisoning.

✖ Yogurt made from unpasteurised milk should not be eaten during pregnancy, as it may contain listeria or other bacteria, which could cause food poisoning.

8 Breastfeeding – the best diet for you and your new baby

Just because your baby has been born, it doesn't mean you can stop thinking about healthy eating. Even if you are not breastfeeding, a balanced diet is important to help your body recover from all the work it's been doing and to replenish the nutrient stores lost during pregnancy. If you are breastfeeding, it is even more important, as the food you eat now will affect the growth and development of your baby. Also, before you know it, your little one will be eating proper food, and, if you have good eating habits, there's a much better chance that he or she will follow suit.

If you found it hard to resist the temptations of ripe Brie or fried eggs while you were pregnant, the good news is that these can go back on the menu. However, small amounts of what you eat will pass into your breast milk, so caffeine and alcohol should still be limited.

Breastfeeding your baby gives the best possible start in life. The list below highlights the many benefits. By paying a little extra attention to your diet, you can improve your baby's chances of a healthy future even more. You can boost brain and eye development and reduce the risk of allergies and asthma.

Breastfeeding gives your baby:

- protection against diarrhoea and gastroenteritis;
- protection against middle ear infections;
- protection against respiratory tract infections;
- a reduced risk of obesity in childhood;
- a reduced risk of diabetes in childhood;
- a reduced risk of allergies such as asthma and eczema.

What's in breast milk?

The composition of breast milk changes in the first few days after birth from colostrum, which is rich in protein and protective factors, to mature milk. It also changes during each feed from foremilk, which is more watery, to hind milk, which contains more calories and nutrients. It even varies with the weather, so that your baby gets more fluids when it's hot, and with the time of day – so your baby really does get just what he or she needs.

On average, breast milk contains about 70 kcal per 100 ml. It is 1.3% protein, 4.1% fat and 7.2% carbohydrate. It also contains omega 3 fatty acids and a range of vitamins and minerals, including B vitamins, vitamins A and E, calcium, iron, iodine and zinc. Breast milk has all the nutrients your baby needs in the first few months of life. It also contains growth factors, hormones and other special proteins, antibodies, white blood cells and nucleotides, which help protect against infection.

It is estimated that if every baby in the UK were exclusively breast-fed for six months, it would halve the number of babies hospitalised for diarrhoea, and the number hospitalised for respiratory infections would be cut by a quarter.

A healthy diet for breastfeeding

A healthy diet while you breastfeed is similar to that for any stage of life. However, there are some things you need to pay closer attention to. When you've just had a baby, it is nice to have things laid down as simply as possible, so the guidelines below should help:

- At least **five portions of a variety of fruit and vegetables** every day. Fruit such as bananas and raisins are especially handy for snacks when you're busy with a new baby.

- **Protein foods**, such as meat, fish, eggs, cheese, beans and lentils.

- **Starchy foods**, such as bread, pasta, rice and potatoes. The extra energy you need for breastfeeding should come from these foods rather than from snacks that are high in sugar or fat.

- **High-fibre foods**, such as wholemeal bread, high-fibre breakfast cereals and pulses. These are particularly important in the early days after having your baby, when constipation is a common problem.

- **Fish** at least twice a week, including at least one portion of oily fish to provide your baby with a good supply of long-chain omega 3 fatty acids.

- **Dairy foods** such as milk and yogurt to supply calcium for your own milk production. This is important for your own health too, as you will have less calcium in your body than normal, no matter how well you ate during pregnancy.

- **Plenty of fluids**. The general advice for people who are not breastfeeding is to drink at least six to eight glasses of fluid a day (approximately 1.2 litres). As you are likely to be producing about 800 ml of milk a day, you obviously need more than this. However, you shouldn't force yourself to drink more than you want. The best drinks are water, milk (skimmed or semi-skimmed) and pure fruit juice.

- **Iron-rich foods**. During the last trimester of pregnancy, your baby accumulates most of the iron he or she needs, at the expense of your iron needs. Your iron levels may therefore be depleted after birth. You will also lose some blood during labour, so it is important to have a good supply of iron when your baby is born. This will replenish your stores and ensure that you have sufficient iron for breastfeeding.

Ten tips for eating well with a new baby

When you have a baby to look after, it can be difficult to think about your diet. However, it is important to make healthy eating and regular meals a priority. This will benefit both you and your baby.

1 Always have healthy snacks at hand so that you don't have to rely on biscuits and buns when you are busy.
2 Don't get into the habit of eating unhealthy take-aways and ready meals to save time. Instead, keep meals simple – you can buy ready-chopped vegetables for a stir-fry, or try one of the almost instant meals listed opposite.
3 Have a big glass of water next to you every time you sit down to feed your baby. When you have a cup of tea or coffee, try to match it with a glass of water.
4 If your baby sleeps in the morning, make yourself a big sandwich with plenty of salad and put it in the fridge for later.
5 When things are going well and you have time to cook, try making extra to go in the freezer.
6 Shop online. If your baby is not a fan of supermarket shopping, Internet shopping can make life much easier.
7 Remember that eating well is more important than how tidy your home is.
8 Try not to graze. Regular eating is important, but it is easy to get into bad habits when you are at home all day. This can result in you putting on excess pounds.

9 When someone asks how they can help, ask them to cook a healthy meal, or suggest that visitors bring fruit instead of chocolates sometimes.

10 Think about whether you are turning to food when what you really need is more sleep, fresh air, exercise or emotional support. If you need help, ask for it (see Resources and useful contacts on page 143).

Ten almost instant meals for busy mums

1 A baked potato filled with tuna, low-fat mayonnaise and some salad.
2 Baked beans on toast, and a glass of orange juice.
3 Vegetable soup and a wholemeal roll.
4 A bowl of cereal with chopped banana or strawberries.
5 Mashed sardines on toast.
6 Peanut butter (or almond butter) and grated carrot sandwich.
7 Low-fat cheese on toast with sliced tomato.
8 Grilled chicken or salmon, couscous and vegetables.
9 Greek salad in wholemeal pitta bread.
10 Pan-fried steak and tomato sandwich.

Do you still need supplements?

Women who are breastfeeding are advised to take a supplement containing 10μg of vitamin D every day. This is because rickets, which is caused by vitamin D deficiency, appears to be re-emerging in the UK. You may have started taking vitamin D supplements during pregnancy, but if not it is a good idea to begin now. If you are eating a well-balanced diet, then you should not need any other supplements.

How your diet affects your milk

Some components of breast milk are affected by the food you eat. The protein and carbohydrate content doesn't seem to vary with a mother's diet, but some studies have found that the fat content can be altered. If you have a low-fat diet and low fat stores, the amount of fat in your breast milk is reduced.

The levels of different fatty acids in your diet also affects the amounts of fatty acids in your breast milk. Women who eat more butter have been found to have increased levels of saturated fat in their breast milk, and women on macrobiotic diets have lower-than-expected levels of saturated fat. In addition, women who never eat fish have much lower levels of EPA and DHA (omega 3 fatty acids). A study of more than 300 women in the Netherlands found that those consuming organic dairy products and meat had higher levels of conjugated linoleic acid (CLA) in their breast milk. CLA is thought to have many health benefits, including boosting the immune system and having anti-inflammatory effects.

By eating one or two portions of oily fish a week, you can boost the levels of omega 3s in your breast milk. This can have beneficial effects on your baby's brain and eye development. Breastfed babies of mothers with higher intakes of long-chain omega 3s have been found to score better on developmental tests, including those for hand and eye coordination.

The myth of poor-quality milk
Women sometimes believe that their milk isn't very good. They may even be told they have 'poor-quality milk'. In reality, the composition of breast milk is unlikely to vary so much that it affects your baby's feeding pattern or immediate growth, unless you are severely malnourished. It is much more likely that your baby's

positioning and attachment while feeding need attention. If you are concerned about your milk supply and are thinking about giving your baby the odd bottle or switching to formula completely, don't rush into it. Make sure you first talk to your midwife or health visitor or call one of the breastfeeding helplines (see Resources and useful contacts on page 143). They should be able to offer you plenty of advice on establishing good breastfeeding.

Yummy – garlic milk

The foods, spices and drinks you consume while breastfeeding directly affect the flavour and odour of the milk you produce. Your baby has already been exposed to a variety of flavours before he or she was born, via the large quantities of amniotic fluid he or she swallowed in the womb. Now your baby is continuing to learn about the great variety of flavours available.

You might think that garlic milk would put a baby off feeding, but this doesn't seem to be the case. It is known that garlic transfers into breast milk – the odour has been detected by scientists, who report that it is at its strongest two hours after garlic is eaten – but babies seem to like it. In fact, babies have been found to stay at the breast longer, suck more often and consume more milk when their mother has eaten garlic.

Another great advantage of flavoured breast milk is that it prepares babies for weaning and enjoying a varied diet in later life. Breastfed babies are less likely to become fussy eaters. A greater acceptance of different flavours is apparent right from the beginning. A number of studies have found that babies exposed to particular flavours, including carrot juice, aniseed and garlic, while breastfeeding are more likely to enjoy the taste later when they are weaned.

Weight loss

It is important to take a balanced and sensible approach to losing weight after you've had a baby. It is not a good idea to lose 3 stone in two months, as Catherine Zeta-Jones was reported to have done. Equally, you can't expect breastfeeding to make the pounds melt away if you eat chocolate biscuits by the packet.

Many new mums feel enormous pressure to lose weight after seeing pictures of super-slim celebrity mums. If you have a nanny, a personal trainer and your own chef, you may be able to follow in their footsteps; however, this isn't a recipe for successful breastfeeding or bonding with and enjoying your new baby. Trying to lose weight rapidly will also leave you feeling drained of energy and could mean both you and your baby miss out on some of the essential nutrients you need. It is particularly important that you don't go on any kind of restrictive diet, such as dairy-free or low-carb, without talking to your doctor. It is much better for you and your baby for you to breastfeed, eat a healthy balanced diet and aim to lose the extra pounds or stones slowly.

It is estimated that breastfeeding requires about 500 kcal per day. You probably need double this if you are feeding twins. During pregnancy, fat stores are laid down to supply some of that extra energy. The amount of additional calories you need while breastfeeding will depend on how much fat you have stored. If you are thin, it's important to make sure you consume plenty of extra calories. You should make regular meals and snacks a priority, to ensure that you and your baby are getting all the calories and nutrients you need. However, if you are overweight, then it is important to concentrate on eating the nutrient-rich foods recommended on page 117, while limiting your intake of high-sugar and high-fat foods.

If you have a very low-calorie diet, your milk supply will be affected. However, if you do have extra pounds to lose, then slow weight loss won't adversely affect your milk. Research has shown that when women lose 1–2lb a week through healthy eating and regular exercise, the amount and quality of their breast milk are not affected, and nor is their baby's weight gain. Eating more high-fibre and low-GI foods can help you lose baby weight at a healthy rate, without feeling so hungry (see page 33).

Although breastfeeding can help you lose weight, not every woman who breastfeeds sheds the pounds effortlessly. Breastfeeding certainly uses up energy, but many breastfeeding women are hungrier and eat more than non-breastfeeding mothers. One study found that weight loss in the six months after birth was related more to a desire to lose weight than to breastfeeding or bottle-feeding. So, if you want to lose weight, don't think that breastfeeding is the solution no matter what you eat. Research into losing weight after giving birth has found that using both diet and exercise together is more effective than either dieting or exercise alone.

Tips for successful weight loss

- Rather than short bursts of physical activity, such as a workout once a week, aim for regular exercise such as walking every day.

- Try to establish regular eating habits. It is all too easy to snack if you're overtired and spending more time at home.

- Try getting some support by joining a slimming club that is suitable for breastfeeding mums, or just meet other mums for a long walk.

- Do exercise that fits into your new lifestyle. It may be easier to go walking with your baby, or get an exercise DVD to do at home, rather than finding someone to look after your baby while you go to the gym or an exercise class.

- Try not to eat on the run. It is much more satisfying to have a sit-down meal and eat slowly; you will then be less likely to overeat.

- If you are having trouble shifting the pounds, make a note of everything you eat for a few days. This may reveal that you are eating more than you thought, and it will show you where you can make some changes.

Foods to avoid when you're breastfeeding

There aren't any foods you need to avoid completely when breast-feeding, but the following should be consumed in limited amounts:

- Don't have more than two portions (140g each) of **oily fish** each week. This is because oily fish, such as salmon and sardines, contain traces of pollutants, which can pass into your breast milk (see page 97).

- Avoid having more than one portion of **shark**, **swordfish** or **marlin** a week.

- Try not to have too much **caffeine**. You may feel in need of a strong cup of coffee, especially if you haven't slept well, but bear in mind that caffeine passes into breast milk, so it won't just be you who enjoys the stimulant effect. Also, babies can't metabolise caffeine as easily as adults can, and so caffeine can build up in your baby's system. There is no specific caffeine limit for breastfeeding, but following the guidelines set for pregnancy would be sensible. Caffeine also makes you dehydrated, so it is important to have plenty of drinks without caffeine as well in order to keep your fluid levels up.

- **Alcohol** should be drunk only occasionally as, like caffeine, it passes into breast milk. It is recommended that you don't have more than 1 to 2 units once or twice a week. You may have heard that alcohol, particularly beer, is good for breastfeeding, but I'm afraid that this has been tested and shown to be a myth (see page xviii).

Research has shown that drinking even small amounts of alcohol reduces the amount of milk women produce and affects breastfeeding. An experiment found that when women consumed orange juice containing 1 to 2 units of alcohol, they produced significantly less milk than when they had plain orange juice. Studies into the amount of milk babies consume after their mother has had a drink have also produced significant results. One study looked at the number of sucks the baby made in the first minute of breastfeeding. It was found that the suck rate was 15% greater when mothers had consumed 1 to 2 units of alcohol; however, the babies were found to consume 30% less milk. It seems that the babies had to work much harder to get milk when their mother had been drinking. It could be that alcohol affects the mother's milk letdown (release of milk to the nipple area). Curiously, babies don't seem to be put off by the smell or flavour of alcohol in the milk, which seems to be strongest 30 minutes to an hour after drinking. Babies given expressed milk from a bottle consume just as much when it contains alcohol as when it doesn't.

In the long term, having the odd drink is not likely to affect the amount of milk your baby takes. Although babies consume less in the 4 hours after alcohol is drunk, they appear to compensate to some extent 8–16 hours later by consuming more milk. However, drinking alcohol while breastfeeding can have other effects. Alcohol may make mothers feel sleepy, but it actually makes babies more restless and they spend less time in 'active sleep'. Also, in the long term, it can affect a baby's well-being. Regular drinking (one drink or more per day) has been found to adversely affect a baby's motor development.

- Most women can eat **peanuts** while breastfeeding. However, if your baby has a parent or sibling with a food allergy, asthma, eczema or hay fever, then avoiding peanuts could reduce the chances of your baby developing a peanut allergy.

- Some **herbs** are traditionally thought to dry up a woman's milk supply. These haven't been tested scientifically, but it might be sensible to avoid taking large doses of sage, mint or parsley while breastfeeding. Use in normal cooking is fine.

Planning a night out

If you are going out and will be having a drink, it is best to plan your feeding beforehand. Alcohol clears from your breast milk at about the same rate as from your blood (just over 2 hours per unit). However, it varies slightly according to your weight. For example, if a 9-stone woman drank 6 units of alcohol, it would take about 14 hours to clear from her milk, whereas an 11-stone woman would clear the same amount in about 13 hours.

The level of alcohol in your milk isn't affected by feeding, so 'pumping and dumping' is unnecessary. It is best to express enough milk before you start drinking to last your baby until the alcohol has completely left your system.

Women are sometimes advised to avoid orange juice, garlic, spicy meals or other foods while breastfeeding. Although it may be sensible to skip a very hot curry when you've just had a baby, generally there is no need to limit your diet 'just in case'. You can eat as normal and just look out for any adverse effects. Possible reactions to food include general upset or restlessness, a rash, runny nose, wind, diarrhoea and explosive nappies.

If your baby has green bits in the nappy, it is probably not because he or she has consumed something they shouldn't have. More likely, your baby has not been getting enough of the nutrient-rich hind milk that comes later during a feed after the watery foremilk.

This sometimes happens because the baby is switched from one breast to the other before he or she has a chance to get the good stuff. If you are worried about the appearance of your baby's stools, talk to your midwife or health visitor.

Sometimes your baby may be upset by something you have eaten, but it is hard to identify the food responsible or determine whether it was something completely unrelated. The section below on colic lists some of the foods most commonly thought to upset babies. Sometimes babies are allergic to specific proteins in the food you are eating. This is not common but is worth considering. An allergy to dairy foods is the most commonly talked about problem, and women may be advised by alternative and complementary therapists to cut out milk and dairy foods from their diet – sometimes without good reason. Only 0.5% of exclusively breast-fed infants have allergies to cows' milk protein, and there are many other reasons why babies suffer from problems such as eczema, diarrhoea and discomfort.

If you have eaten something that you suspect doesn't agree with your baby, then you could try avoiding the food for a week, before trying it again. If the same thing happens, you might be better steering clear of it for a while. However, it is important that you don't cut out whole food groups, such as dairy foods or foods containing wheat, without talking to your midwife, health visitor or doctor. If you do, both you and your baby could be missing out on essential nutrients.

Colic

It can be very distressing if your baby has colic, and you are probably willing to give anything a go. However, before you start avoiding dairy foods, wheat, soya, eggs or any other food, it is important to learn as much as you can about colic and to talk to your midwife, doctor or health visitor. Sometimes improving your baby's position when feeding can make a real difference. If not, try not to worry unduly. Although feeding is unlikely to be enjoyable and relaxed for either of you, babies with colic generally take just as much milk as others and gain weight normally.

What is colic?
Colic is thought to affect about one in five babies. It is characterised by periods of frantic crying at roughly the same time every day, typically in the early evening. A baby with colic is also likely to draw their knees up to their chest, pass wind and become red in the face. Colic generally appears in the first few weeks and disappears by the time a baby is 3 or 4 months old. If you are unsure whether your baby has colic, it is best to talk to your doctor to rule out other possible causes of distress.

Colic and cows' milk

In some babies, colic may be the result of lactose intolerance or an allergy to cows' milk. These may sound very similar, but they have quite different causes and should be treated differently.

Lactose intolerance

This is a sensitivity to the sugar (lactose) found in milk, including formulae and breast milk. If a baby doesn't produce enough of the enzyme lactase, he or she is unable to break down the lactose sugar in the small intestine. The lactose therefore passes into the large intestine, where it is fermented, producing hydrogen and methane gases and discomfort. If your baby is receiving formula, your health visitor may suggest switching to a lactose-free or low-lactose formula. Breast milk contains lactose irrespective of what you eat, so cutting out milk and dairy foods from your diet won't help: your body will still produce lactose for your milk. What you can do, however, is give your baby lactase, for example Colief®. This shouldn't be given to your baby directly but should be added to a small amount of expressed milk. Your baby can then be given the milk from a spoon or cup, before being put to the breast as normal for a feed. The problem is often called 'transient lactose intolerance', because babies generally grow out of it. Once your baby is 3 to 4 months old, he or she should be producing sufficient lactase to digest the lactose so you won't need to supply additional lactase.

Allergy to cows' milk

This is an immunological response to the proteins that the milk contains. These are found in most formula milks, as these are based on cows' milk. The proteins are also present in breast milk if the mother consumes cows' milk or any dairy products such as yogurt and cheese. If your baby is receiving any formula, then switch to a hypoallergenic variety. The only way to ensure that your baby does not receive cows' milk proteins from your breast milk is to remove all cows' milk products from your diet. Your doctor or health visitor will be able to advise you on how to do this, and how and when to try re-introduction, possibly in a clinic.

Other causes and cures

In reality, there is usually no cure for colic. However, several strategies may help to ease the symptoms of colic. No one really knows the cause of most cases of colic, but some research suggests that the baby's immature digestive tract could have difficulty coping with milk; as a result, the baby suffers from cramps. Colic may also be due to the baby swallowing air bubbles when he or she feeds or cries. To help minimise this, try to sit your baby as upright as possible during feeding rather than lying him or her flat on their back, and burp your baby well. The drug simeticone may also help; this is an anti-flatulent, which changes small bubbles of air in your baby's intestine into larger bubbles that are easier to burp up. Simeticone has been used for years and is readily available from pharmacists, for example as Infacol®. It may also help if you breastfeed your baby on the same side until he or she has definitely had enough milk; switching from one breast to the other before your baby's got enough of the high-fat hind milk may mean that he or she feeds more to compensate, meaning that your baby has a larger volume of milk to cope with and more lactose than he or she can handle comfortably.

Sometimes women find breastfeeding so stressful with a colicky baby that they are tempted to stop. You may even wonder whether your baby would do better with a bottle of formula. However, research has shown that formula-fed babies are much more likely to get colic than those who are breastfed.

Adapting your diet may help to relieve your baby's colic symptoms. Different things seem to affect different babies, but it may be worth cutting out certain foods to see whether the colic is reduced. It is best to try just one dietary change at a time, otherwise you could end up eating a very limited diet and missing out on some nutrients. If, after a week, there is no improvement, go back to your normal diet. If your baby's symptoms get better, then it might be worth skipping the food for a while, if it is something you can live without, such as tea or onions. However, if it is a key food, such as fish or dairy products, then you should try gradual re-introduction or look for alternative sources of the nutrients that you will be missing. It may be that you just need to eat less of the trigger food, or to eat it in a different form. For example, if milk is the problem, you may find that if you have a smaller amount of milk, or consume milk as part of another cooked dish, then it is OK.

Here are the foods most commonly suspected of causing or aggravating colic:

- tea and coffee;
- alcohol;
- cruciferous vegetables such as broccoli, cauliflower and cabbage: these may encourage the production of wind;
- cows' milk and milk products, such as cheese and yogurt;
- wheat and corn;

- fish;
- eggs;
- onions;
- chocolate;
- citrus fruit.

The whole area of diet causing adverse effects in breastfed babies is quite complicated, and guidelines are still evolving. Whether it is colic or some other unwanted symptoms, it really is best to get professional help from your GP, health visitor or state-registered dietician.

What about me?

Most of this chapter has focused on how breastfeeding affects your baby, but breastfeeding also benefits you:

- It stimulates the uterus to contract back to its pre-pregnancy size.
- It reduces the risk of breast cancer.
- It reduces the risk of ovarian cancer.
- It increases the chances of losing weight and returning to your pre-pregnancy weight.
- It gives you some protection against osteoporosis.

Eating well while you are breastfeeding is important not only for your baby but also for your own health and well-being. If your diet is less than ideal, you could suffer, even if your baby is fine. Research has shown that mothers can have signs of malnutrition, including bone demineralisation, B vitamin deficiencies and multiple infections, even while their breastfed babies appear healthy, show no signs of malnutrition and have a normal or low-normal weight. So, by all means congratulate yourself if your baby is thriving, but don't forget that how you are doing is important too. As well as improving your physical health, eating well can make you feel better. It will boost your energy levels and could even help with post-natal depression.

Although there is not much research into post-natal depression, having a good intake of zinc and vitamin B_6 could be important. In addition, intake of DHA and EPA is thought to affect mental health. Several studies have looked at whether higher intakes of these long-chain omega 3s can prevent or treat post-natal depression, but the results are inconclusive, with only some studies finding a benefit. However, given the other benefits, it may still be worth ensuring that you have a good intake of DHA and EPA.

9 Preparing for another pregnancy

If you are starting to think about having another baby, or planning for your first, then this is the ideal time to get your diet and general lifestyle in order. A healthy balanced diet is important before as well as during pregnancy. What you eat now can have an enormous impact on your chances of getting pregnant and of having a healthy baby.

If you can make dietary improvements before you become pregnant, they will have a much bigger effect than if made later. So, rather than burning the candle at both ends while you still have the chance, use this time to get into shape and give your baby the best possible start in life. Taking even just a few steps in the right direction can help. And as your family grows, you will all reap the health benefits of good dietary habits.

You are unlikely to know you are pregnant for about two weeks after you conceive, so it is worth erring on the side of caution when it comes to food safety. That means avoiding excess alcohol and caffeine and thinking more about food hygiene. If this is your first pregnancy, or you need reminding about just what to eat for pregnancy, then the pre-pregnancy checklist overleaf will help, but you may also find Chapters 1 and 2 useful. Then, when you get a positive pregnancy test, you can celebrate without worrying and feeling guilty about what you have eaten or drunk over the past few weeks. Also, you can ensure that your body has a good store of nutrients in case you suffer from morning sickness and don't feel like eating much in early pregnancy.

The pre-pregnancy checklist

Do

- Try to reach a healthy weight.
- Take a supplement containing 400 μg of folic acid. This is important in the very early days after conception before you know you are pregnant and will reduce your risk of having a baby with spina bifida or a neural tube defect.
- Eat a healthy balanced diet.
- Be careful about general food hygiene (see page 22).
- Exercise to keep fit and relieve stress, but avoid rigorous exercise programmes as these can reduce fertility.
- Talk to your doctor if you are taking any prescription drugs or herbal medicines.
- Relax and make the most of life. You may get pregnant straight away, but it could take some time. Stress reduces fertility and there won't be much time for relaxing once your new baby arrives.

Don't

- Drink alcohol. It can cause birth defects and increase the risk of miscarriage. If you do decide to drink, stick to no more than 1 to 2 units once or twice a week and avoid getting drunk. Your partner should cut down too: not only for moral support, but because even moderate drinking can lower his sperm count.

- Eat liver or take supplements such as cod liver oil, which contain high levels of vitamin A.

- Eat shark, swordfish or marlin, and don't have more than two tuna steaks or four cans of tuna a week. Traces of mercury in these fish can affect your baby's nervous system.

- Eat peanuts if you have a family history of allergies.

- Drink too much coffee, tea and other drinks containing caffeine.

- Smoke or take recreational drugs such as cannabis.

Why weight matters

Your weight before you get pregnant can affect your fertility and your baby's health. If you are unsure whether your weight is appropriate for your height, you can find out by using the graph on page 14 or working out your BMI (page 13). Being underweight can make it more difficult to conceive and increases the risk of miscarriage in the first trimester (three months) of pregnancy. It can also increase the risk of your baby having a low birth weight and being unwell.

Being overweight can also reduce your fertility. A study in Denmark found that obese couples were three times more likely to have trouble conceiving compared with couples of a normal weight. Being over-weight also increases the risk of complications during pregnancy, in-cluding infections, high blood pressure, pre-eclampsia and diabetes, and the risk of birth defects, including heart and limb deformities. An-other problem is that being overweight makes it more difficult for your midwife to monitor your baby during pregnancy and labour, and there is a greater chance of problems arising during the birth.

Don't be unduly concerned if you are overweight or underweight. These are risks, not certainties, and they are intended to show why it is important to reach a healthy weight. At the same time, you are in an ideal position now to do something about it and to increase the chances of everything going well.

Still carrying weight from your last pregnancy?

Mothers who don't manage to lose the weight they gained in their first pregnancy increase the risk of complications when they become pregnant again. A Swedish study of more than 150 000 women found that even small weight gains could be a problem. Women who gained just 1 or 2 BMI units following their first pregnancy (around 6–12 lb) were 20–40% more likely to go on to suffer from high blood pressure or gestational diabetes than those who retained less weight. Gaining more than 3 BMI units presented further problems, increasing the risk of stillbirth by 60% and the risk of pre-eclampsia by more than 70%.

The risks weren't only increased in women who became classified as overweight or obese following their first pregnancy. They also applied to women who were still classified as normal weight but who had gained weight. If you are one of the many mums affected by lingering baby fat, then you need to make some long-term changes to your diet and physical activity. To start with, why not get your little one in the pushchair, by the hand or on a bike and head for the park – it'll do you both some good.

How do you measure up?

If your BMI is under 20, you are underweight. To increase your BMI, you should eat larger quantities but still try to have a healthy diet. If you have only a small appetite, then choose more energy-dense foods such as full-fat dairy products, nuts, seeds and avocados. You could also use more vegetable oils in cooking or salad dressing. If you find large meals daunting, then don't worry – just eat small snacks throughout the day. If you do a lot of exercise, it might also help to reduce your workouts. In order to have a regular menstrual cycle and normal ovulation, women need to have a reasonable amount of body fat (at least 22%). Yours may be below this if you have a heavy exercise schedule. If you find it difficult to increase your body weight, then talk to your GP about getting some help, particularly if you have a history of eating disorders.

If your BMI is between 20 and 25, you are a healthy weight for your height. However, if you are right at the very bottom or very top of the range, you should keep an eye on your weight, and likewise if you gained weight following your last pregnancy (see the box opposite). Otherwise, you don't need to worry, and you certainly shouldn't think about losing weight in anticipation of putting it on when you get pregnant: research has shown that women who do this could be putting themselves at increased risk of premature delivery. Instead, you should make sure that you eat a healthy diet in order to get all the nutrients your body needs.

If your BMI is over 25, you are overweight. You need to make some changes to your diet and increase the amount of physical activity that you do. You may be keen to get on with the business of baby-making, but don't try losing weight too quickly. Strict dieting will deprive your body of the essential nutrients it needs and can actually reduce rather than increase your fertility. Restrictive diets such as the low-carb Atkins diet may seem like a good idea – some people certainly achieve phenomenal weight loss with this kind of eating. However, research suggests that low-carb diets reduce your chances of becoming pregnant. If you currently follow the Atkins diet, you should stop before trying to get pregnant and instead follow a more balanced diet.

It is best to make long-term changes to your eating habits so that you can achieve a slow but steady weight loss of one or two pounds a week. This can be done by cutting down on fatty and sugary foods and increasing your intake of fruit and vegetables, high-fibre foods and water. At the same time, you should take more exercise. Trying to incorporate more walking into your everyday life and using the stairs more often will also help.

Of course, losing weight is easier said than done, but what better incentive is there? By shedding the pounds now, you should feel better, increase your fertility, have an easier pregnancy and birth, and have a healthier baby. If you find weight loss difficult, particularly if you have a lot of weight to lose, then talk to your GP or join a reputable slimming club that doesn't promise instant success but encourages healthy eating and long-term results.

If you are very overweight, it is worth holding off trying to get pregnant until after you have managed to lose some of the extra pounds. Then you will have a better chance of everything going well. If you are less overweight, there shouldn't be any problem with you trying for a baby while you lose up to two pounds a week, providing you do it through sensible healthy eating and exercise.

What is a healthy diet?

A healthy diet when trying for a baby is basically the same as at any other time. It includes at least five portions of fruit and vegetables every day, plenty of starchy foods such as bread and rice, and some good sources of protein and calcium, such as meat, fish, pulses, milk and dairy foods (see page 7). Folic acid is another key nutrient for pregnancy. As well as taking a supplement, try to increase your intake of folate-rich foods such as oranges and broccoli.

If it isn't long since your last pregnancy or you have recently stopped breastfeeding, then healthy eating now is especially important, as your stores of key nutrients, including vitamins A and D and omega 3s, may be low. In addition, up to half of young women have a low iron store, which puts them at risk of anaemia in pregnancy. By building up your iron stores now, you can prevent this happening (see page 45).

Fertility foods
Adopting a 'fertility diet' could boost your chances of getting pregnant, according to researchers at Harvard University. In a study of more than 17000 women trying for a baby, they found that those with certain dietary habits and lifestyles were less likely to suffer fertility problems.

The 'fertility diet' pattern they identified was characterised by:

- a high consumption of monounsaturated fats rather than trans fats, e.g. consuming olive oil, nuts and seeds and avoiding processed foods such as cakes and biscuits;

- eating more vegetable protein than animal protein, e.g. avoiding large amounts of meat and eating beans and lentils instead;

- having plenty of low-GI (glycaemic index) carbohydrates rather than high-GI ones, e.g. wholegrain cereals and oats instead of white bread and cakes;

- eating a moderate amount of full-fat dairy produce rather than only low-fat versions of products such as milk and yogurt;

- consuming plenty of vitamins and iron from plant foods and supplements.

They also found that cutting down on alcohol and caffeine was important, as were controlling weight and having a reasonable level of physically activity. When they looked at infertility due to ovulatory disturbances, which is one of the most common problems, they found a 70% lower risk among women following the diet most closely.

Slugs and snails or sugar and spice

If you already have a boy or two, and think that a little girl would now be the icing on the family cake, is there anything you can do to achieve your ambition? There is certainly plenty of advice out there about what to eat to get the girl or boy you want, but can what you eat really determine the sex of your baby?

It is not guaranteed, but it may be possible to slightly sway the odds. One theory holds that eating certain foods alters the pH of the vaginal environment, making it more hospitable to X (female) or Y (male) sperm. It seems that X sperm prefer more acidic conditions, while Y sperm fare better in alkaline conditions. Some believe that the crucial factor is the ratio of sodium and potassium to calcium and magnesium in your diet. If you want a boy, then you need to consume more sodium and potassium, so foods such as meat, sausages and other salty meat products, bananas, rice and pasta are recommended. At the same time, you need to cut down on calcium- and magnesium-rich foods such as milk and dairy products, ice cream, nuts, pulses, chocolate, spinach and wholemeal bread. If you're dreaming of all things pink, however, you should do the opposite – consume less salt and more milk and chocolate.

Another theory, based on animal experiments, suggests that fat intake is crucial to sex selection. For years, scientists observed that animals in the wild were more likely to have male offspring if they were fed well. Researchers altered the fat intake of experimental mice to see how it affected their offspring. They found that mice with diets high in saturated fat were twice as likely to produce male babies as female babies. Mice on a low-fat, high-carbohydrate diet, by contrast, were more likely to have females babies.

On the whole, when it comes to diet and sex selection, it is probably wiser to leave it to fate. The suggested dietary manipulations are not particularly good for you or your baby, whatever sex they turn out to be. Consuming lots of salt or saturated fat or restricting your intake of certain minerals is unhealthy and certainly not ideal when trying for a baby. In any case, at best, the diet can only slightly alter your chances of conceiving a child that is the 'right' sex. Some experts put the success rate at about 50%, i.e. the same as doing nothing. Alternatively, you could look at methods that don't involve manipulating your diet, such as only having sex at certain stages of your menstrual cycle or changing sexual positions. These are based more firmly on scientific principle and have a better chance of success. To conceive a girl, it may help to have frequent sex after menstruation but to abstain for two or three days before and after ovulation. For a boy, avoid sex in the days before ovulation, and ejaculation deep into the vagina is advised.

A little extra – should you take supplements?

If you are healthy and eating a balanced diet, there should be no need to take supplements, apart from folic acid, which all women should take when trying to conceive. However, if you have been trying for a baby for some time without success, evidence suggests that a multivitamin and mineral supplement may help. Make sure you choose a supplement that is specifically formulated for pre-conception and pregnancy. Also, think of it as a safeguard for days when you are very busy and can't eat as well as you should: a supplement is not a substitute for healthy eating.

Having trouble conceiving?

If you haven't become pregnant as quickly as you had hoped, try to relax. Some couples find that they conceive their first baby very easily, but second time around it takes longer than expected. This is called secondary infertility and appears to be a growing problem. It may be because women are delaying motherhood until fertility levels are starting to drop anyway, and they are then that little bit older when they try for number two. Also, having already had a baby, women may be more relaxed and less worried about eating 'fertility foods' or having sex at the right time of the month.

If you are trying to get pregnant either for the first time or to expand your family, don't get frustrated. This may be easier said than done, but the statistics may comfort you: although you may not be in the 50% of couples who conceive within two or three months, you could be among the 85% who manage it within a year. Before suspecting more complex problems, make sure you address simpler issues such as your weight. Research has shown that both underweight and overweight women increase their chances of conception when they gain or lose weight, respectively. You may feel happy with your current weight, but making the necessary changes, so that your BMI is within the 20–25 range, could save you going through difficult, possibly expensive, fertility treatment.

An unhealthy lifestyle may not seem to harm some women's chances of getting pregnant. But for others, it can be enough to tip the balance. So, as well as addressing any weight issues, look carefully at every aspect of your diet, including your intake of alcohol and caffeine. As mentioned above, supplements may also help. In addition, you might like to look at your intake of vitamin B_6, which is found in fish and certain nuts and vegetables. A study of Chinese textile workers found that low intakes of vitamin B_6 reduced the chances of conception.

Of course, diet isn't everything. Don't overlook the obvious issues, such as having regular sex around the time of ovulation. Your partner can optimise his fertility too by improving his general health. If you both need to make lifestyle changes, then you can support each other. If you need more advice, the baby charity Tommy's has an excellent guide to pre-pregnancy, which is available free (see Resources and useful contacts on page 142). If you are still worried or have been trying to get pregnant for more than a year without success (or more than six months if you are over the age of 35), then talk to your GP.

Resources and useful contacts

Association of Breastfeeding Mothers

Counselling hotline plus information about local breastfeeding clinics, support groups and baby cafes.

www.abm.me.uk
Helpline: 08444 122 949 (9.30 a.m. to 10.30 p.m.)

Breastfeeding Network (BfN)

Drop-in support clinics and helpline.

www.breastfeedingnetwork.org.uk
Helpline: 0844 412 4664 (9.30 a.m. to 9.30 p.m.)
Drugline: 0844 412 0995 (for information about taking prescription drugs while breastfeeding)

Centre for Pregnancy Nutrition, University of Sheffield

Information on healthy eating and food safety before and during pregnancy and while breastfeeding.

www.shef.ac.uk/pregnancy_nutrition
Helpline: 0845 130 3646

Cry-sis

Support for families coping with excessively crying and demanding babies.

www.cry-sis.org.uk
Helpline: 08451 228 669 (9 a.m. to 10 p.m.)

Healthy Start

Government scheme providing free supplements and food vouchers for pregnant women and mothers of young children on a low income.

www.healthystart.nhs.uk

La Leche League

Local support groups and helpline with calls being taken by mothers in their own homes.

www.laleche.org.uk
Breastfeeding helpline: 0845 120 2918 (any time)

National Breastfeeding Helpline

Helpline funded by the Department of Health and staffed by trained volunteer mothers from the Breastfeeding Network and the Association of Breastfeeding Mothers.

Lines are open 9.30 a.m. to 9.30 p.m. every day of the year to offer support and practical advice on all aspects of breastfeeding.

Helpline: 0844 20 909 20

NCT (formerly the National Childbirth Trust)

Organises antenatal classes and provides advice and local support for pregnancy and early childhood.

www.nctpregnancyandbabycare.com
Pregnancy and birth helpline: 0870 444 8709
Breastfeeding helpline: 0870 444 8708

NHS Direct

Lots of useful information on the website about pregnancy, breast-feeding and general health, including symptoms of various illnesses.

www.nhsdirect.nhs.uk
Information line: 0845 4647 (24 hours a day)

TAMBA (Twins and Multiple Births Association)

Information and support network for parents of multiples.

www.tamba.org.uk

Tommy's

Provides a range of free books and leaflets about pre-pregnancy and pregnancy and advice on particular problems such as pre-eclampsia and toxoplasmosis.

www.tommys.org
Information line: 0870 777 3060

Vegan Society

Provides information for vegans.

www.vegansociety.com
Tel: 0121 523 1730 (9.30 a.m. to 5 p.m. Monday to Friday)

Vegetarian Society

Charity providing information and advice on all aspects of vegetarian-ism. Provides good information sheets on pregnancy and weaning and also provides recipes.

www.vegsoc.org
Tel: 0161 925 2000 (8.30 a.m. to 5 p.m. Monday to Friday)

If you have been given *The Pregnancy Book* by your doctor or midwife, you will find lots of other useful contact details at the back of that.

Index